FEMINIST COMMUNITY RESEARCH

FEMINIST COMMUNITY RESEARCH
Case Studies and Methodologies

Edited by Gillian Creese and Wendy Frisby

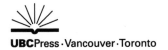

UBCPress · Vancouver · Toronto

20 19 18 17 16 15 14 13 12 11   5 4 3 2 1

Printed in Canada on FSC-certified ancient-forest-free paper that is processed chlorine- and acid-free.

Library and Archives Canada Cataloguing in Publication

Feminist community research : case studies and methodologies / edited by Gillian Creese and Wendy Frisby.

Includes bibliographical references and index.
Issued also in electronic format.
ISBN 978-0-7748-2085-1 (cloth); 978-0-7748-2086-8 (pbk)

   1. Communities – Research. 2. Feminist theory. I. Creese, Gillian Laura II. Frisby, Wendy Mae

HM756.F46 2011	307.072	C2011-905357-8

e-book ISBNs: 978-0-7748-2087-5 (pdf); 978-0-7748-2088-2 (epub)

Canadä

UBC Press gratefully acknowledges the financial support for our publishing program of the Government of Canada (through the Canada Book Fund), the Canada Council for the Arts, and the British Columbia Arts Council.

This book has been published with the help of a grant from the Canadian Federation for the Humanities and Social Sciences, through the Aid to Scholarly Publications Program, using funds provided by the Social Sciences and Humanities Research Council of Canada.

UBC Press
The University of British Columbia
2029 West Mall
Vancouver, BC V6T 1Z2
www.ubcpress.ca

Contents

Preface and Acknowledgments

This collection of essays on feminist community research marks the thirty-fifth anniversary of Women's and Gender Studies (WAGS) at the University of British Columbia.* Although UBC is a research-intensive university that is internationally renowned for more traditional approaches to research, our community of feminist scholars receive much less attention and are often isolated in their own departments and by disciplinary boundaries. Feminist community research (FCR) remains, quite simply, under-profiled and under-supported at many academic institutions, even though much of it is on the cutting edge of interdisciplinary, collaborative, and policy-oriented research that is increasingly being called for by numerous constituents, including post-secondary educational institutions that are seeking to strengthen relationships between universities and various communities.

---

* Women's and Gender Studies at the University of British Columbia is made up of two administratively separate but functionally interlinked units. An undergraduate program in the Faculty of Arts administers a major and minor in women's and gender studies. The Centre for Women's and Gender Studies (CWAGS), located in the College for Interdisciplinary Studies, administers graduate programs and has more than ninety affiliated faculty associates and research associates. The first undergraduate courses were offered in 1973, thirty-five years before we began this book in 2008. An undergraduate major in women's and gender studies was launched in 1991, the same year the centre was founded. Graduate programs followed, with an MA in 2000 and a PhD in 2001.

This book provides an opportunity to highlight a variety of feminist community research conducted by researchers associated with Women's and Gender Studies at UBC and their colleagues and community members. Authors who conduct feminist community research were invited to contribute original essays to the present volume. At least one author of each chapter is connected to Women's and Gender Studies at UBC through a formal affiliation as a faculty member, current or former graduate student, or a faculty or research associate. Some chapters' authors are also members of various communities engaged in FCR, including formerly incarcerated women, Aboriginal women, peer outreach sex workers, women from rural communities, and recent immigrants. Other authors represent partner community organizations such as the BC Centre for Excellence in HIV/AIDS, Sex Workers United Against Violence Society, Umoja Operation Compassion Society/African Family Services, Whitevalley Community Resource Centre, and WISH Drop-In Centre Society. Within the University of British Columbia, authors are located in diverse disciplines and interdisciplinary units, including the Centre for Women's and Gender Studies, the School of Community and Regional Planning, the Department of Educational Studies, the Human Early Learning Partnership, the School of Human Kinetics, the Faculty of Medicine, the School of Nursing, the Department of Sociology, and the undergraduate program in Women's and Gender Studies. There is also one author each from the Department of Sociology and Anthropology and the Faculty of Science at Simon Fraser University; as well as one each from the Department of Nursing at Trinity Western University, Child, Family and Community Studies at Douglas College; the Department of Social Work at Northern Lights College; and the Department of Educational Policy Studies at the University of Alberta. Collectively, this diversity in authors represents a range and breadth that contributes, we hope, to the advancement of understanding what feminist community research can and should be.

This book is a collaborative enterprise that brings together a collection of FCR projects in dialogue with each other, rather than a simple collection of discreet solicited chapters. In keeping with the collaborative aims of feminist community research, the authors worked together for over a year in an effort to ensure that the chapters would "talk to one another" in a variety of ways. We are providing details about our writing process in this preface because we found it to be much more stimulating and rewarding than the traditional approach of writing independent chapters without ever having discussions with other authors. Our collaboration, which was geographically facilitated by the fact that at least one author of each chapter is affiliated with UBC, included an initial meeting at which authors talked about their visions for the book and for their own chapters, developed guidelines for working together, and established timelines. Authors then drew on a set of common questions, developed collectively, that were intended to help orient our thinking and writing, while providing common threads throughout the collection. These questions were:

1 What feminist methodological and/or ethical issues are addressed in the FCR project?
2 What challenges were involved in doing FCR?
3 What research strategies (both successful and unsuccessful) are documented for readers?
4 What do *community* and *reflexivity* mean in the context of the FCR project?
5 In what ways are issues of social justice, policy, and/or social change embedded in the research?

Chapter drafts were subsequently uploaded onto a website so we could read each other's work.

In the spring of 2009, we held a one-day symposium where authors presented their chapter drafts and received feedback from each other. We challenged each other, asked thought-provoking questions, and encouraged each other to explore creative ways of presenting our ideas (e.g., by drawing on autobiographical narratives, conducting comparisons across more than one FCR project, and conducting research across geographical borders). Revised chapters were then submitted and another round of feedback was provided through an author peer review process before chapters were submitted to UBC Press for external review.

We gratefully acknowledge the feedback provided by authors and reviewers that helped us sharpen and deepen our arguments, while creating synergies across chapters. The collegial and collaborative chapter-writing process is helping to create a stronger community among this group of FCR researchers at, or connected to, UBC, and we feel privileged to be a part of it. Although many of us have links to the same university, we seldom have had the chance to talk to and learn from each other in this way. It is hoped that the supportive and stimulating opportunity for mutual learning that resulted from writing this book will foster additional productive collaborative efforts in the future, while contributing to the feminist methodology literature with a social justice agenda.

We also very gratefully acknowledge the contributions made by various community members whose voices are heard throughout this collection, the funders who supported the various feminist community research projects reported upon, the research assistants who helped us conduct the research, the organizations that partnered in the research, and the significant others in our lives who support our humble efforts at trying to make a difference. We owe thanks to the Women's and Gender Studies program for providing seed money for this publication, and to the Centre for Women's and Gender Studies for funding the conference. We also owe a great debt to the team at UBC Press, especially to our editor, Darcy Cullen, to Emily Andrew, Anna Friedlander, members of the Publications Board, and the anonymous reviewers for their very helpful advice. Finally, we want to thank Wynn Archibald and Jane Charles, our administrative support team at Women's and Gender Studies, whose efforts routinely go above and beyond anything we have a right to expect. We both feel incredibly privileged to be part of a collegial and supportive environment at Women's and Gender Studies that provides a welcome oasis in a broader institutional environment that too often undervalues the kind of feminist community research profiled in this volume.

Gillian Creese and Wendy Frisby
Vancouver, British Columbia
11 August 2010

FEMINIST COMMUNITY RESEARCH

1

Unpacking Relationships in Feminist Community Research
Crosscutting Themes

WENDY FRISBY AND GILLIAN CREESE

Feminist community research (FCR) uses innovative methodological approaches to tackle complex social problems faced by those who are rarely included in knowledge production and policy making. This approach, and the present collection, is timely because it comes at a moment when there are calls for increased collaboration between universities and communities to generate knowledge that is widely distributed and that contributes to improved social policies. All research, not just FCR, is socially embedded knowledge generated from "somewhere," located in specific institutional arrangements and relations of power and privilege that structure the social world. The authors in this book intentionally set out to problematize the social embeddedness of processes of knowledge production. They do so by critically reflecting on their own feminist community research, while simultaneously searching for new ways to develop better collaborative research relationships across diverse communities, all with the aim of producing knowledge that will contribute in some way to creating a more just society.

Negotiating Contested Relationships

The key underlying theme woven through all the chapters in this volume is the multiple and ongoing ways that contested relationships must be negotiated as part of feminist community research processes. The nature of relationships with other researchers, community collaborators, community organizations, research assistants, funders, and others involved in the research influences whether particular research even takes place, affects how the research unfolds and what gets accomplished, and ultimately determines who benefits from the research (and who does not). Yet, academics and the partners and communities they work with receive little if any training on how to build trusting and mutually productive relationships that avoid, or at least minimize, the numerous and serious potential pitfalls that can arise when insufficient resources and skill are devoted to building and sustaining diverse feminist community research relationships.

We have yet to uncover a book dedicated to the topic of *negotiating contested relationships in feminist community research,* and this is where the fundamental contribution of the book lies: in ferreting out the many tensions involved in research relationships; in analyzing rather than glossing over what went well, as well as what did not; in sharing the lessons learned so that others might benefit from our successes and our mistakes; and in considering the consequences of negotiating contested relationships for all those involved. Hence, one aim of this book is to share new strategies that emerged in the ongoing and never-ending search for more respectful and ethical approaches to conducting feminist community research.

All of the chapters in this volume examine research that falls under the broad heading of feminist community research. However, it is important to acknowledge at the outset that the authors depart from varying theoretical perspectives and name their approaches in a variety of ways that speak to the different emphases in their work. For example, different authors call their work participatory action research, community-based research, community health research, capacity-building research, or post-colonial research. At the same time, regardless of the specific methodological terms the authors use, every piece in this collection is informed by debates in feminist methodologies. Gender figures prominently in each analysis, but as the different chapters demonstrate, gender is inextricably tied to other axes of power and privilege, including race, social class, colonial histories, sexuality, age, and other forms of oppression that have a profound influence on the knowledge claims made (Collins 2005; Razack 2002; Reid and Frisby 2008). The authors are also all engaged in research with communities of various kinds and are committed, in one way or another, to research oriented towards social change. The definitions of *community* and the methodological strategies used vary considerably across the chapters, spanning local, diasporic, and global contexts, while simultaneously problematizing related methodological dilemmas.

There is a long tradition of feminist methodological writings that draws our attention to the important but contentious issues of negotiating research relationships. The unequal power relations, contested notions of truth and knowledge, building knowledge based on lived experience, ethical issues involved in working with funders and partners while representing the "Other," and the politics of voice and representation in meaning making are particularly relevant to research in this collection (Ramazanoglu and Holland 2002; Brooks and Hesse-Biber 2007; Fonow and Cook 2005; Harding 2004). As politically engaged feminist researchers, we all struggle to some degree with Donna Haraway's (1991) "greasy pole" – the dilemma of simultaneously critiquing notions of objectivity and knowledge claims that silence the communities we engage with, while maintaining a focus on social change that requires convincing "real world" accounts that will influence policy makers and others to take up the research findings in relevant ways.

The starting point for feminist community research is acknowledging that our own knowledge claims are historically situated, socially embodied, and mediated through multiple and shifting relations of power and privilege. Engaging in reflexivity that opens up negotiations over what knowledge claims can be made, by whom, for what purpose, and within what frames of reference is difficult and often uncomfortable (Ramazanoglu and Holland 2002). As Linda Tuhiwai Smith (1999) points out, research is never "innocent," and learning to share in processes of knowledge creation is a precondition to decolonizing research methodologies. Most feminist researchers (ourselves included) still have much to learn about what more equitable "sharing" in knowledge creation might mean, while acknowledging our "epistemic responsibility" (Skeggs 1997) as critical scholars. To varying degrees, the authors in this collection also grapple with the tensions between critical and poststructuralist approaches that fundamentally challenge the limits of our quests to tell fuller or less partial feminist truths (Houle 2009; Visweswaran 1994).

Feminist community research takes up these issues and attempts to do research differently to disrupt dominant frameworks, disciplinary silos, and taken-for-granted assumptions that maintain the status quo. Those engaged in FCR attempt, however partially, to transcend colonizing research relations, bring to the surface voices that are often excluded from knowledge production and policy making, and critically reflect upon how it can all be done better (Frisby, Maguire, and Reid 2009). Above all, FCR questions what is at the centre and what is at the margins of knowledge making by illuminating the tensions and considering the alternatives. Therefore we hope this book will represent one contribution to a larger discussion on the role of feminist research "with" (rather than "on" or "for") different communities (Ristock and Pennell 1996).

As is true in most qualitative research, the research process is embedded in developing relationships of various kinds. FCR involves the complicated negotiation of relationships with community – individual community members and/or community-based organizations – as well as with funders, university research ethics boards, and often government-based policy makers. The dynamic nature of how relationships evolve across very different social locations is a central theme in the chapters in this book. Some of the benefits, limitations, and tensions that arose are explored in discussions of different types of relationships. These include relationships between, for example, clinical researchers and inmate participants, university-based researchers and immigrant service organizations, white (male and female) feminist researchers and racialized researchers and community members, middle-class researchers and women living in poverty, and sex workers as peer researchers. The complicated web of relationships necessary to conduct this type of research becomes even more apparent when one considers the negotiations that must occur within and between researchers, community members, community partners, funders, institutions, and government officials who may be involved in the research. Every layer of these relationships is saturated with differences in power, access to resources, and control over meaning making. The negotiations that take place sometimes produce constructive tensions leading to new insights, but they may also threaten to undermine the very enterprise of transformative knowledge production.

Collectively, in the chapters that follow, we strive to unpack central methodological dilemmas encountered in our own attempts to negotiate relationships in feminist community research. We do this not to undermine the value of this work, but rather to share lessons learned with others interested in engaging in FCR as one way of fostering transformative action and social change, both large and small, intended and unintended (Reid, Tom, and Frisby 2006). We want to foster hope in both the relevance of and the possibilities for this type of research, while at the same time signalling the serious pitfalls that need to be carefully negotiated in order to avoid naive or even harmful research, no matter how well intentioned. Hope becomes evident when all parties involved in FCR talk about the positive impact that it has had on their lives, even for a moment, despite the ongoing struggles involved in doing the research and the persistent and pervasive material and structural conditions that oppress people's lives on a daily basis. In the absence of such hope, we may remain content either to let the academy conduct unethical research that damages relationships or forgo doing research altogether. Neither of these alternatives is inspiring. Those breaking new paths in feminist community research, such as the authors of this book, are harbingers for hope in both the academy and the broader social world. As a result, our imperfect achievements in this area merit celebration.

Crosscutting Themes

There are a number of crosscutting themes related to negotiating contested relationships that link this collection together. The FCR projects examined here grapple with a range of different substantive topics such as community capacity building, health care, international development, caregiving, poverty, and immigration. Running through these substantive topics are a number of methodological themes related to negotiating relationships. These themes include deconstructing concepts and categories, reflexivity, voice and representation, the importance of time and place, the political economy of FCR, ethics, emotions, and efforts at fostering social change. Below, we draw your attention to how we see the crosscutting themes providing the threads that link the chapters together. The aim here it not to (re)create an FCR orthodoxy; rather, it is to raise critical questions that should be carefully negotiated with community members and partners to develop projects that are responsive to the diverse people who take part in them.

Deconstructing Concepts and Categories

The chapters that follow go some way in unpacking a wide variety of concepts, including *community, giving voice,* and *postcolonialism,* and raise questions about multiple meanings and the consequences of using static and sometimes binary terms. Meanings of community in this book are wide-ranging. For some, community means a specific group of women at a certain time and place, even though it is acknowledged that these groups are never homogeneous. For others, community means working with organizations like immigration services or connecting communities based on geography (e.g., rural and urban) or similar experiences (e.g., living on social assistance). And for others, it means creating community for women who are often isolated from one another (e.g., sex workers or former prison inmates).

Other terms, like *reciprocity, transparency, reflexivity,* and *agency,* are common in FCR, but we need to ask what these terms really mean for the different people involved. What are the limitations, tensions, and (un)intended consequences in trying to live up to the ideals associated with these terms, and how do understandings and practices of these concepts shift over time, especially when community membership in FCR changes because of attrition or the addition of new members? To illustrate, Joan Anderson asked in one of our author meetings what using terms like *marginalization* and *vulnerable people* does to the agency of those with whom we engage? It is by deconstructing and reconstructing categories and approaches collectively that new possibilities for doing FCR emerge.

In many different ways, the importance of locating women's experiences in colonial histories and the ongoing impact of colonial relations is raised, as in the chapter by Joan Anderson, Koushambhi Basu Khan, and Sheryl Reimer-Kirkham. This leads to questions about the concept of *post-colonialism*, given the continuing weight of colonial systems of oppression. Several of the chapters highlight the different ways in which colonialism provides a context for understanding findings in feminist community research with Aboriginal women and with immigrants from various locales around the world.

Reflexivity

The goal of reflexivity is a central element of feminist qualitative research methodologies (Ramazanoglu and Holand 2002; Smith 1999), one that is embraced by all the authors in this book. Reflexivity involves interrogating how differences in power and privilege shape research relationships in diverse contexts. In many chapters, unconventional means of sharing power and resources were successfully pursued, such as when Paul Kershaw was able to reroute research funding directly into the hands of a community organization. In another example, Jill Chettiar, Mark Tyndall, Katharine Chan, Devi Parsad, Kate Gibson, and Kate Shannon worked with survival sex trade workers to interview others in similar situations to better understand the issues around the prevention of HIV infection. Yet, power sharing is often stymied by the rules of funders, partnering organizations, research ethics boards, and the privileges that many researchers carry with them – even as they try to unpack those privileges. This was particularly evident in Tara Gibb and Evelyn Hamdon's chapter, where they interrogate how the organization that commissioned their study exerted control over the research questions that differed from the questions that immigrant women themselves thought were important. Several authors engaged in discussions with community members about who gets to define *knowledge* and for what purpose, leading to new ways of thinking about what research questions should be asked and what constitutes adequate answers. It is, in part, by engaging in collective reflexivity that capacity can be built for future projects.

Voice and Representation
Many of the chapters in this collection grapple in different ways with related questions of whose voices get heard and who speaks for whom in feminist community research. For example, at our authors' symposium, we learned that women in prison were not allowed to be named as co-authors on one of Ruth Martin's previous publications, thereby preventing the voices of women inmates from being heard. In another example, Gillian Creese, Xin Huang, Wendy Frisby, and Edith Ngene Kambere discuss how translation can imperil voice and how participants with stronger English-language skills can have their voices privileged over others in FCR.

Place and Time
Feminist community research draws attention to the importance of time in relationship building by raising questions about how the research is tied to past histories as well as to future actions that may or may not occur as a result. Connecting with people over time illustrates the fluidity of relationships and interpretations of one's circumstances and points to the limitations of one-time cross-sectional methodologies in illuminating complex social issues. Penny Gurstein, Jane Pulkingham, and Silvia Vilches specifically ask how we account for the silences connected to attrition in FCR over time through multiple interviews. Time and place also figure into who gets recruited to participate and who does not, as the most isolated members of a community are the least likely to take part.

The politics of place are also apparent. Some Aboriginal community members in the capacity-building project with Colleen Varcoe, Helen Brown, Betty Calam, Marla Buchanan, and Vera Newman wanted to talk with researchers in the natural environment, in connection with which an Aboriginal woman talked about the tensions of speaking about the research in a fancy hotel in downtown Vancouver. Others, like Leonora Angeles in her chapter, point to the conflicts inherent in conducting FCR in a university setting, and conversely, the challenges of travelling repeatedly to places inhabited by community members who are in remote locations around the world. Conducting research with immigrants who are now living in geographies new to them becomes complicated when other members of FCR research teams have not been to the countries from which the immigrants have come, raising questions about how such researchers can interpret and make sense of stories of relocation.

The Political Economy of FCR

Several authors in this volume address the tensions and politics involved in managing budgets, when the requirements of funders do not match up well with the funding needs for FCR. At our authors' symposium, which was described in the preface, Jane Pulkingham framed this tension as the "political economy of FCR," which entails negotiating the competing demands of funders, university financial officers, and diverse communities, as well. Unequal power relations are imbued in the allocation of FCR budgets: it is often university-based researchers who use their privilege to leverage funding, while within the confines of funder regulations, having power over disbursements. For example, some funders will not allow child care expenses to be covered, even though having adequate child care is often a prerequisite for parents to take part in FCR. Another important consideration is that community partners and university-based researchers are on salary with their employers while conducting the research, but community members are sometimes expected to volunteer their time or receive small honoraria, thus exacerbating unequal power relations. This can result in a mentality of "cash for quotes," as Colleen Varcoe aptly pointed out at our authors' symposium, raising questions about just how voluntary participation really is (or is not) in some FCR projects. It is important to consider how honoraria and other forms of payment can be coercive and exploitative, even when designed to lessen power imbalances by compensating participants for their time and contributions to the knowledge-production process.

Ethics

Ethical research is at the heart of searching for better ways to conduct feminist community research to minimize potentially exploitatative research processes or outcomes that could be harmful in some way. Many of the chapters in this volume address ethics in terms of being responsible to participants and community partners by developing processes and relationships that are collaborative and more transparent. Some chapters illustrate the disjuncture between ethical review standards required by funders and universities and how this can create significant barriers to FCR. Colleen Reid, Pamela Ponic, Louise Hara, Robin LeDrew, Connie Kaweesi, and Kashmir Besla relay an account of a community that wished to be named in publications, and an ethics board's refusal to permit that to happen, thereby undermining the agency of research participants and the likelihood that the research would contribute to social change in ways that they had envisioned.

Emotions

Those engaged in feminist community research are not concerned with maintaining objectivity and distant relationships with study participants. In fact, friendships are often forged, and sometimes broken, over the course of the research, as expectations shift and can or cannot be met. A whole range of emotions are felt over time by research participants (including researchers), ranging from elation to despair, happiness, anger, hope, and disappointment. Shauna Butterwick's autobiographical account fleshes out the emotions tied to research relationships with women living in poverty and how her own position of privilege at times both assisted and hindered the actions taken. Another example appears in the dialogue between Ruth Martin and Kelly Murphy, in the chapter they co-authored with Marla Buchanan, as they chart their changing responses to each other over the course of their relationship, first as physician and prison inmate, and later as co-researchers. Both of these chapters document how emotional responses, judgment, and personal pain can lead to new insights and/or create barriers to meaning making.

Policy and Social Change

Conducting research that contributes to progressive social change concerns all the authors in this book, and many chapters contribute to a rethinking of specific social policies – such as social assistance regulations, prison reform, public recreation policies, literacy programs, development initiatives, health care delivery, and settlement services. If social change is the goal of feminist community research, an important question to ask is how do we get policy makers to listen to this type of research in an appropriate way, especially when we engage in the type of self-critique that can serve to undermine it? We contend that by continually deconstructing categories and approaches, possibilities for reconstructing them become apparent.

Collectively, this volume raises important implications in terms of the politics of knowledge production, policy making, and social justice. Although the main focus is on methodology and the micro-politics of doing FCR, the analyses point to significant gaps between community members' lives and the assumptions underlying public policy. Rather than positioning policy makers as the villains whose rules negatively affect women's lives, we recommend considering forming strategic alliances with "policy champions," where appropriate, by incorporating them into FCR from the outset. An example of this is outlined in the chapter by Gillian Creese, Xin Huang, Wendy Frisby, and Edith Ngene Kambere, where the authors describe a workshop that brought recent immigrant Chinese women together with forty policy makers from different levels of government as part of the FCR study design. It was clear that some of the policy makers were very committed to making change but had few opportunities to engage directly with those for whom they were supposed to be developing policy, and they encountered considerable constraints that are important to identify and try to work around when advocating for policy change.

One suggestion for future research could include policy-mapping projects that illustrate the intersecting consequences that multiple policies have on people over time, how this can further their marginalization, and how different policies could lead to more equitable outcomes. It is by paying attention to all of these crosscutting themes that are crucial to negotiating relationships in feminist community research that the potential for having a positive policy influence is enhanced. At the same time, while this book covers a wide range of topics and types of communities, many other groups, issues, and contexts could not be covered. As a result, this volume represents a starting point that needs to be built upon by further research and policy development.

Organization of the Book

Following this introduction, the book begins with two chapters that raise broad questions about postcolonial feminist research and capacity building in international contexts. The focus then turns to a series of distinct local case studies that take up various dimensions of these issues. The book ends with two chapters that grapple with the thorny issues of ethics and knowledge production, followed by brief reflections by the editors.

In Chapter 2, "Community Research from a Post-Colonial Feminist Perspective: Exemplars from Health Research in Canada and India," Joan Anderson, Koushambhi Basu Khan, and Sheryl Reimer-Kirkham compare how social relations are organized through different histories of colonization in different geographical areas. Drawing upon examples from their independent FCR with women who are Aboriginal; women who have immigrated to Canada from India, Hong Kong, and China; women who are Canadian-born of European descent; and women who live in the slums of

Delhi, India, they compare the relevance of post-colonial feminist theory in community health research. While acknowledging some of its limitations, their analysis demonstrates how post-colonial feminist theory provides a lens for identifying structural and historical forces that sustain gendered power relations that are reflected in inequitable access to health care.

In Chapter 3, "Feminist Demands, Dilemmas, and Dreams in Introducing Participatory Action Research in a Canada-Vietnam Capacity-Building Project," Leonora Angeles picks up on the complexities of conducting international FCR involving globalized university-community partnerships. Capacity-building projects provide one foundation for realizing the dreams of FCR in terms of transforming communities. Angeles's project on Localized Poverty Reduction in Vietnam, however, demonstrates the ways in which research relationships are constrained by institutional and bureaucratic practices that are embedded in gendered hierarchies and lines of authority, constraints that are compounded by international partnerships.

In Chapter 4, "Travels with Feminist Community-Based Research: Reflections on Social Location, Class Relations, and Negotiating Reciprocity," Shauna Butterwick provides an autobiographical account of her research relationships with a group of local women living on low incomes. In particular, she explores the unexpected ways that reciprocity can occur in FCR. As she aptly points out, "there is welcome recognition of the responsibility of universities *to* non-academic communities, but little commentary on social class and other forms of difference such as gender and race that profoundly shape social relations."

In a novel approach to FCR, Chapter 5 documents how a team of women who are survival sex workers were hired and trained to play an active role in guiding and developing a research project designed to indentify and fill gaps in information on the prevention of HIV infection and harm reduction services for women. In "Voices from the Street: Sex Workers' Experiences in Community-Based HIV Research," Jill Chettiar, Mark Tyndall, Katharine Chan, Devi Parsad, Kate Gibson, and Kate Shannon problematize the strategy of using "peer researchers" and contemplate the impact that their project has had on community members who live in an area with high concentrations of drug use and survival sex work.

A comparative analysis of how research relationships are further complicated appears in the account by Gillian Creese, Xin Huang, Wendy Frisby, and Edith Ngene Kambere of conducting FCR with immigrants. In Chapter 6, "Working across Race, Language, and Culture with African and Chinese

Immigrant Communities," they compare and contrast what *community* meant in two different research projects, and they document the strategies used and struggles encountered in working across difference. They also reflect on how the relationships that evolved in their respective FCR projects affected the interpretation of the data, given the politics of meaning making.

In Chapter 7, "Tangled Nets and Gentle Nettles: Negotiating Research Questions with Immigrant Service Organizations," Tara Gibb and Evelyn Hamdon consider the impact of relationships with partnering organizations in FCR. Their analysis details the problems that arise when university-based researchers and immigrant service organizations tackle research questions related to employment but that "miss the mark" because they are not tackling issues identified as being of central importance by new immigrants themselves.

Penny Gurstein, Jane Pulkingham, and Silvia Vilches provide an analysis of how longitudinal interviewing with lone mothers poses implications for neo-liberal welfare policy reform. In Chapter 8, "Challenging Policies for Lone Mothers: Reflections on, and Insights from, Longitudinal Qualitative Interviewing," they examine the strengths, limitations, and dilemmas of doing critical policy-relevant research on poverty based on the lived experiences of lone mothers.

In provocatively titled Chapter 9, "White *Cowboy*, Black Feminism, Indian Stories," Paul Kershaw tells his story about the methodological tensions involved in collaborating with women of colour and Aboriginal women in an FCR caregiving project that placed their expertise at the centre of theory building. He details the collaborative grant-writing process that was undertaken with a partnering organization, the journal writing and interviews that took place, and the challenges encountered given his privileged social location.

Chapter 10, by Ruth Elwood Martin, Kelly Murphy, and Marla Buchanan, titled "Inside and Outside of the Gates: Transforming Relationships through Research," provides yet another important slant on negotiating contested relationships in FCR. The key question they ask is: "How are research relationships reconstituted from the traditional dichotomy of researcher/subject within a prison research project that values collaborative participation, authentic relationships, community, reflexivity, transparency, and transformation?" Undertaking FCR in the largely inflexible environment of a women's prison produced particular tensions that ultimately led to shifting the research focus outside the prison gates.

Ethical issues are front and centre in Chapter 11, "Living an Ethical Agreement: Negotiating Confidentiality and Harm in Feminist Participatory Action Research," by Colleen Reid, Pamela Ponic, Louise Hara, Robin LeDrew, Connie Kaweesi, and Kashmir Besla. The authors outline how their relationships with women living in rural and remote communities were compromised because of the ethical agreement required by the funder of their project. Thus, they add yet another layer to relationship complexity in feminist community research.

Chapter 12 returns to processes of capacity building and ethics, but this time FCR is positioned as a site for mutual learning and decolonizing practices when working with Aboriginal communities. In "Capacity Building Is a Two-Way Street: Learning from Doing Research within Aboriginal Communities," Colleen Varcoe, Helen Brown, Betty Calam, Marla Buchanan, and Vera Newman show how capacity building in conventional research implies that non-academics are somehow deficient. Based on their project, they advocate for new conceptualizations that decolonize research relationships within Western research frameworks.

Finally, in the last chapter, "Reflections: Promises and Limits of Feminist Community Research," we consider some of the lessons learned through these various examples of FCR, highlighting the diversity of feminist approaches, the multiplicity of strategies pursued, and the limits of reflexivity and mediation of power relations that suggests the quest to "get it (at least partially) right" will always be a work in progress.

Concluding Thoughts

This book has several audiences in mind. We hope to speak to other practitioners and students of FCR, or those who are interested in pursuing this type of research in the future, as part of an ongoing conversation on how to create more productive forms of feminist community research. Learning how to work across university-community boundaries in more egalitarian ways is not always easy, especially when FCR involves work with hard-to-reach groups, as many of the chapters in this book illustrate.

The difficulties of developing respectful, responsive, and ethical research relationships are profoundly shaped by the institutional structures in which research occurs. A second audience, then, involves funders, peer reviewers of grants, and university research ethics boards, who may not be familiar with community research or with feminist methodologies more generally. While attempting to protect the rights and integrity of research "subjects," ethical guidelines are too often imposed in a paternalistic and positivistic fashion that undermines the agency of study participants and, hence, the ability to develop more equitable collaborations that reject hierarchical "researcher-subject" relationships.

Although current models of research ethics at play in funding bodies and universities can make more equitable collaborative research difficult, it is precisely this type of collaboration with communities and socially relevant knowledge dissemination that these bodies are increasingly calling for. Thus, it is our hope that sharing our candid stories of the problems, tensions, strategies, and (at least partial) successes that we have encountered in negotiating relationships in FCR will encourage others to engage in more effective FCR projects, contribute to progressive social change, and at the same time, foster a rethinking of ethical and funding guidelines to facilitate more flexible and relevant ways of doing feminist community research.

NOTE

Although we are the authors of this introductory chapter, we acknowledge that many of the points raised here originated in conversations with other authors in this book, as we participated in the collaborative chapter-writing process described in the preface.

REFERENCES

Brooks, Abigail, and Sharlene Nagy Hesse-Biber. 2007. "An Invitation to Feminist Research." In Sharlene Nagy Hesse-Biber and Patricia Leavy, eds., *Feminist Research Practice*, 1-24. Thousand Oaks, CA: Sage.

Collins, Patricia Hill. 2005. *Black Sexual Politics: African Americans, Gender and the New Racism*. New York: Routledge.

Fonow, Mary, and Judith Cook. 2005. "Feminist Methodology: New Applications in the Academy and Public Policy." *Signs* 30(4): 2211-36.

Frisby, Wendy, Patricia Maguire, and Colleen Reid. 2009. "The 'F' Word Has Everything to Do with It: How Feminist Theories Inform Action Research." *Action Research* 7(1): 13-19.

Haraway, Donna. 1991. "Situated Knowledges: The Science Question in Feminism and the Privilege of Partial Perspectives." In D. Haraway, *Simians, Cyborgs, and Women: The Reinvention of Nature*, 183-201. New York: Routledge.

Harding, Sandra. 2004. "Rethinking Standpoint Epistemology: What Is 'Strong Objectivity'?" In Sharlene Nagy Hesse-Biber and Michelle Yaiser, eds., *Feminist Perspectives on Social Research*, 39-64. New York: Oxford University Press.

Houle, Karen. 2009. "Making Strange: Deconstruction and Feminist Standpoint Theory." *Frontiers: A Journal of Women Studies* 30(1): 72-93.

Ramazanoglu, Caroline, with Janet Holland. 2002. *Feminist Methodology: Challenges and Choices*. London: Sage.

Razack, Sherene, ed. 2002. *Race, Space and the Law: Unmapping a White Settler Society.* Toronto: Between the Lines.

Reid, Colleen, and Wendy Frisby. 2008. "Continuing the Journey: Articulating Dimensions of Feminist Participatory Action Research." In Peter Reason and Hilary Bradbury, eds., *Handbook of Action Research: Participative Inquiry and Practice*, 2nd ed., 93-105. London: Sage.

Reid, Colleen, Allison Tom, and Wendy Frisby. 2006. "Finding the 'Action' in Feminist Participatory Action Research." *Action Research* 4(3): 313-30.

Ristock, Janice L., and Joan Pennell. 1996. *Community Research as Empowerment: Feminist Links, Postmodern Interruptions.* Toronto: Oxford University Press.

Smith, Linda Tuhiwai. 1999. *Decolonizing Methodologies: Research and Indigenous Peoples.* London: Zed Books.

Skeggs, Beverley. 1997. *Formations of Class and Gender.* London: Sage.

Visweswaran, Kamala. 1994. "Betrayal: An Analysis in Three Acts" In Inderpal Grewal and Caren Kaplan, eds., *Scattered Hegemonies: Postmodernity and Transnational Feminist Practices*, 90-109. Minneapolis: University of Minnesota Press.

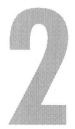

Community Research from a Post-Colonial Feminist Perspective
Exemplars from Health Research in Canada and India

JOAN M. ANDERSON, KOUSHAMBHI BASU KHAN, AND SHERYL REIMER-KIRKHAM

The purpose of this chapter is to consider the directions provided by a post-colonial feminist (PCF) epistemology in community research. It is generally acknowledged that feminist scholarship is underpinned by a common concern with gender, but as McCall tells us, "feminist researchers have been acutely aware of the limitations of gender as a single analytical category" (2005, 1771). Although many scholars now address the complex intersections that organize social relations, the varied epistemological and theoretical approaches to feminist inquiry give rise to different research questions and, hence, to different methodological issues in community research.

This chapter takes us into a new terrain of analysis that cuts across two different geographical regions, each with a different history of colonization, and it is to be read as a work in progress. The chapter is organized into three main sections. We begin with a conversation among the three of us to locate ourselves and our research, and to articulate the post-colonial feminist concepts that we have found most salient in our research. Drawing on exemplars from health research conducted in Canada and India, we discuss how we came to locate our work within a PCF epistemology. Anderson draws on her early research with women who immigrated to Canada from India and Hong Kong/China, some of whom were living with a chronic illness, and Canadian-born women of European descent; Khan's examples are from her work with women living in the slums of Delhi, India; and, Reimer-Kirkham's examples are from research in an Aboriginal community, as well as ethnographic studies in Canadian hospitals situated in ethnically and religiously diverse communities. We then elaborate on the central concepts in PCF scholarship and offer a post-colonial feminist critique of community and community research. But no theory is without its critics. So, in the section following, we problematize the notion of post-colonialism in the contexts of Canada and India – the countries in which our research studies were conducted. We conclude by examining the intersection of theory, methodology, and methods through a PCF lens with the aim of explicating what PCF scholarship has to offer to community-based research.

Locating Our Work in Post-Colonial Feminist Epistemology and Identifying Salient Concepts

To a large extent, our social and political location determines the questions that we are drawn to investigate and how we engage in the process of knowledge production. As Joseph reminds us, personal and professional biographies play "a crucial part in the construction and representation of knowledge" (2009, 12). Two of us were born and grew up in countries that were colonized and gained independence "from foreign rule." We now make Canada our home, but we are among those often referred to as "immigrant women of Colour."[1] The third woman was born in Canada of Euro-Canadian descent within a religious diasporic community. We bring these biographies to our intellectual work, but we did not begin our research journeys as "PCF scholars." We, therefore, address the following two questions in our conversation: How did we come to PCF scholarship, and what insights from these theories inform our work?

How We Came to Post-Colonial Feminist Scholarship

Anderson

My journey began in my research with immigrant and Canadian-born women who were living with a chronic illness. In my early research, my aim was to understand the cultural meanings that shaped women's management of their illness. But, through women's narratives, I learned that although cultural meanings were important to them, culture intersects in powerful ways with a complex set of social relations, located in women's histories and their position in the Canadian labour market.

Compared with Canadian-born women, many immigrant women participating in my early research did not speak English,[2] limiting the jobs that were available to them. But they had no time to learn English. Many worked long hours *to make ends meet.* Including overtime, some of these women worked twelve-hour days, six days a week, and then went home to mind the children and do the housework. *Economic survival was paramount.* Although these women were determined to make the most of their lives, their testimonies brought into sharp focus the harsh realities of everyday existence.

I came to understand that women's life circumstances, not static cultural beliefs, shaped illness management – the positioning of women from "Third World" countries in the workforce reflects deep structural issues, which are mostly glossed over. [3] My interpretive lens shifted from essentializing women's cultures to focusing, instead, on material context (Anderson, Blue, and Lau 1991). These were not just theoretical insights; they had profound policy and practice implications. The issue became one of understanding the contexts of women's lives, and then how to address structural inequities and deliver equitable health care.

Reimer-Kirkham

I, too, realized the inadequacies of culturalist approaches and the need for critical interpretive frameworks early in my scholarly career. As I interviewed nurses about caring for "culturally diverse clients" for my graduate thesis (Reimer-Kirkham 1998), I noted a profound disjuncture between nurses' accounts of racism and the multicultural discourses that predominated at the time. In a subsequent study of intergroup relations in health care, post-colonial theory provided less ideological ways to understand racializing practices at individual and institutional levels, particularly in identifying structural forces that sustain uneven relations of power (Reimer-Kirkham 2003; Reimer-Kirkham and Anderson 2002). Post-colonial theory drew attention to how discourses of who "belonged" in health care (reflected in sentiments such as "Why don't they learn English? This is Canada") echoed colonial constructs of a hegemonic White centre and marginalized Others along linguistic, racialized lines.

A recent participatory action research project with an Aboriginal community highlighted fundamental questions about the processes and purposes of Western research, and the very real risks of re-inscribing colonizing histories through the research process (Smith 1999). Although members of the university-based research team had partnered with the Aboriginal community for more than a decade in the context of nursing education, and the research project was welcomed by the community's health committee, questions regarding our desired "partnership" layered on to historical colonial relations and operated as subtext throughout the project. Understanding colonial histories, decolonizing research approaches, and respecting indigenous knowledges became important pursuits for mutually satisfying research.

Khan

Growing up in Delhi and having spent considerable childhood time in the company of "domestic helpers," who were women from nearby slums, I have always been keen to understand their everyday struggles, challenges, and their "small victories." However, in my early works I tended to focus on gender and poverty issues alone and ignored the role of history. I did not adequately realize the ways in which the dominant discourses about slums, primarily the stereotypical and stigmatizing images, organized the lives of these marginalized women. With time and engagement in critical literature, particularly post-colonial feminist literature, I came to appreciate how history shapes people's lives and makes them more vulnerable to different forms of marginalization. I became aware that dominant discourses about slums and slum dwellers (usually migrant labourers) could be traced to India's colonial past, when migrants from states neighbouring Delhi were viewed as the "Other" – the illiterate, jobless, poor, "polluting" people of low caste and status who represented a threat to Delhi's urban growth and whose presence led to urban policies that (until recently) were geared towards demolition and the resettlement of slum dwellers in the outskirts of the city (Vedeld and Siddham 2002). Engagement with women, and listening to their stories, made me realize the need for an intersectional analysis that accounts for the social, economic, and cultural, as well as the historical, factors influencing their lives. It prompted me to question the taken-for-granted assumptions and stereotypes about slum populations and the need to disrupt the mainstream dominant discourses.

What Insights from Post-Colonial Feminist Theories Informed Our Work?

Anderson

It was not until I had read the writings of Patricia Hill Collins (1990) and other scholars such as Trinh (1989), Mohanty (2003), Brewer (1993), hooks (1984), and Bannerji (2000) – the writings of PCF and black feminist scholars – that I began to understand how various social relations that are historically inscribed, and socially reproduced, intersect to shape not only the illness experience, but also our varied experiences and opportunities in everyday life. While the concept of *intersectionality* is now pivotal in critical feminist research, we must credit the writings of scholars such as Patricia Hill Collins (1990) and Rose Brewer (1993) for developing an analytic perspective that illuminated the varied experiences of women, and the simultaneity of different forms of oppression. Through these writings, I came to locate my research in both post-colonial theorizing and in black feminist epistemology: *post-colonial black feminist* scholarship appropriately describes the theoretical direction that now informs my work.

I tend not to draw a sharp distinction between black feminist epistemology that has come out of the scholarship of black feminists in the United States and Britain and post-colonial feminist writers, for example, Narayan (2000) and Gandhi (1998). While I acknowledge the different histories and contexts that have shaped the lives of women from different parts of the world, slavery, colonization, and neo-colonization contribute to a shared struggle. Furthermore, I use the term *black* as it is used by scholars such as Himani Bannerji (2000) to denote a politics of coalition, rather than shades of skin colour.

Reimer-Kirkham

Further insights from PCF and indigenous epistemologies that stand out for me have to do with critical reflexivity and the construction of identity, particularly as a White woman in regard to conducting research with Aboriginal peoples and non-European Canadians. Aboriginal scholars such as Smith (1999) and Battiste, Bell, and Findlay (2002) alert me to the very real possibility of complicity in the ongoing colonizing potential of research. Post-colonial theorizing has amplified this concern about representation with the question, Can the subaltern speak? Spivak's probing question, the subject of her essay with that title (1988), has focused attention on issues that are core to any PCF endeavours concerning "representation and essentialism; the relationship between the First-World intellectual and the Third-World object of scrutiny" (Bahri 2004, 199). Such questions provide a cogent check for Western and/or White researchers, such as myself, prompting self-reflexivity regarding (mis)representation and colonizing research, while also creating opportunity for strategic alliances where points of connection are made along multiple axes of difference for the purposes of promoting social justice. With post-colonialism's focus on *race* and the accompanying trajectories of colonial practices, reading my own identity as a White woman through a racial lens (Frankenberg 1993) positions me to consider how advantage and disadvantage operate, and how oppressor and oppressed are not essentialized categories of Other and Us but, rather, coexist deep within each (Lorde 1984).

Khan

Following my engagement with post-colonial feminist literature, I came to recognize, besides the importance of our positioning in history, the multiple intersecting identities that each one of us may adhere to at any point in time. It enabled me to understand, in the context of slum women's lives, that "there is no pure site of identity organized around a single axis" (Gedalof 1999, 2) but, rather, a woman's identity and her positionality could be seen as the "meeting point" between various social institutions, discourses, and practices. Concepts like diaspora space (Brah 1996), against purity (Gedalof 1999), borderlands (Anzaldua 1987), and cultural hybridity (Bhabha 1994) particularly informed my work, as they helped me to understand the unique social fabric of slums, which could be viewed as a mix of village life and that of the anonymous city. These concepts made me appreciate the ways in which slum women's lives got shaped by discourses that are problematic and gendered and that both constrained and facilitated the choices that women made that, in turn, had a critical influence on their health. Post-colonial feminism encouraged me to contest fixed notions of either urban city or village life and to understand the culturally hybrid space (Bhabha 1994) that gets created in the slums.

Post-Colonial Feminist Scholarship: Salient Themes and How PCF Informs the Notion of Community

We elaborate here on some of the salient points introduced in our conversation that, we suggest, are central to PCF scholarship, and we then discuss how post-colonial feminist scholarship informs the notion of *community*. The themes of race and racialization, particularly in the context of other intersecting oppressions, are undoubtedly some of the more obvious foci of PCF scholarship. Acknowledging the centrality of these themes, a PCF reading makes evident how such relations of power are embedded in and operationalized through history and place. More than a deconstructive tool, PCF creates space in a constructive manoeuvre for agency of subaltern and subjugated knowledges. It is these two complementary capacities of PCF that we highlight here, as salient themes, and apply first to a critique of the concept of multiculturalism and then to community-based research (CBR).

History and Place Matter

The influential writings of early post-colonial scholars emphasize that we are all positioned in history; they examine how the processes of colonization, and the knowledges produced, underpinned and continue to underpin hierarchies of knowledge and who is constructed as the inferior "Other" and who has the right to produce knowledge. These ideas operate as subtexts to shape life experiences and opportunities, as Phoenix (2009) has so eloquently described, in her use of diaspora and post-colonial theory to examine the ways in which women who, as children, had immigrated to the United Kingdom from the Caribbean experienced racialization.

Post-colonialism, as a term, has been applied variously – as historical epoch, global condition, geographical location, method of scholarly inquiry, or even as current impossibility – but shared across these applications is a concern with historical and contemporary continuities of colonization and decolonization in specific places and specific times. An examination of the Canadian and Indian contexts relevant to our research illustrates how colonization proceeded in different places, namely, the specificity and locality of post-colonialism.

Locating Canada within post-colonialism is itself a conflicted exercise. Canada is often understood as an invader-settler nation, with a history quite different from other colonized countries. Williams and Chrisman (1994), for example, point to the problem of including White settler colonies such as Canada, New Zealand, and Australia under the category of post-colonial, particularly because they were not subject to the coercive measures suffered by actual colonies and because of their current position in global capitalist relations. Others positing a post-colonial Canada focus on Canada's process of establishing nationhood apart from Britain and her Commonwealth as a decolonizing process, a conception itself critiqued as exclusionary and racist in its imagining of Canada as a White bicultural society of English and French speakers (Moss 2003). These interpretations, however, overlook First Nations experiences of historical neo-colonialism, whereby indigenous peoples have through the centuries been decimated by assimilationist policies that have taken away land, health, and the basics of physical, social, and psychological survival. Indeed Battiste (1998) and Battiste, Bell, and Findlay (2002), among other scholars, tell us that Aboriginal peoples in Canada continue to suffer the effects of colonization through the suppression of their knowledge, epistemologies, and languages; and they call for decolonizing practices to right these injustices. Historically, the Canadian state has enacted a series of devastating policies characterized by assimilation, domestication, and wardship with the creation of reserves, the appropriation of Aboriginal lands, the forced removal of children into residential schools, discriminatory attitudes towards Aboriginal people, and a continued lack of vision in terms of the effects of health, social, economic, and political disparities (Adelson 2005; Browne 2007). In this sense, a claim to Canada as "post-colonial" can be disputed in light of the situation of ongoing internal colonialism for Aboriginal peoples.

Post-colonialism in the Indian context presents somewhat of a contrast to the Canadian context. India was an invaded colony with a clear demarcation between the colonizers and the colonized in terms of language, culture, and "race," and there was a specific date when the colonizers "left" and India achieved its "freedom." Colonialism, then, in the context of India almost invariably "becomes a question of periodization" (Mani 1990, 29), as it does seem like a thing in the past. This is not to ignore that India is very much a part of the global economy and that multinational corporations are equally operative in India, nor to suggest that Indians are unaware of the cultural and ideological "influence" (or imposition) of the West. In fact, a close examination reveals the continued influence of the West in a dominant position in many contexts within India, including in the writing of Indian history itself. Chakraborty (1992) notes how Europe works as a silent referent, with Indian history being merely a variation of the master narrative, namely, "the history of Europe." In this sense "Indian" history assumes a subaltern position. It is against this background of European dominance that all historical knowledge gets produced in India and, in that sense, Indian history will always appear as a "mimicry of a certain 'modern' subject of 'European' history and is bound to represent a sad figure of lack and failure" (Chakraborty 1992, 350).

Based on these examples of Canada and India, we see how a post-colonial feminist framework draws attention to the importance of history and place as structuring social relations. Reflecting the range of ways in which "post-colonialism" resonates for various groups, Brydon notes that revisiting "historical memory is necessary for Indigenous, settler, and immigrant populations alike, but operates differently for each" (2003, 53). Indigenous concerns are those of sovereignty and repossession of land, settler interests are typically those of nationhood, and immigrant concerns tend to align with post-colonialism and, we argue, ongoing colonizing processes. Arising from these histories and localities are subjugated knowledges that must be given voice to correct injustices.

Writing in Subaltern Voices and Use of Subjugated Knowledge to Correct Inequities and Injustices

Post-colonial scholarship contests "master narratives" and the notion of a universal standpoint on knowledge production, and it provides a counter-point to knowledges that are produced within dominant Euro-American discourses. Post-colonial feminism unmasks the set of social relations that have silenced the subaltern voice, and it claims a space from which to speak, as illustrated by an example from Indian history: the abolition of *Sati* (Hindu widow sacrifice) in the early nineteenth century. Archival records represent the abolition of Sati as a contest between modernity and tradition, as a struggle between the British "civilizing mission" and "barbaric" Hindu practices, and regard it as the birth of modern India (Prakash 1992). As argued by Mani (1987), the very existence of these historical documents shows how women were seen as the site for the constructions of authoritative Hindu traditions by both the indigenous patriarchy and the colonial powers. The debate left the women with no position from which to speak, that is, the colonized subaltern woman was silenced (Spivak 1985, 1988; Prakash 1992).

Another form of re-inscribing the silencing of women from places such as India has occurred, ironically, within feminist theorizing itself. Women in India, like women all over the globe, experience discrimination that could be traced to an intersection of identity factors such as gender, caste, social class, race, religion, and sexual orientation. These intersecting forces produce complexities that are often unique to the context of India, shared to an extent with other "Third World" women, but remarkably different from Western contexts. It is these complexities that Western feminists need to recognize and create space for Indian (or "Third World") "feminist models of the self" (Gedalof 1999, 51). Complex histories of non-Western societies thus challenge the notion of the ubiquitous all-knowing Western subject (Ahluwalia 2003) and resist master narratives from Western feminist discourses.

The need to give voice to subjugated experience is not limited to non-Western women. Although having different histories, Aboriginal women in Canada and immigrant and refugee women from the "Third World" carry a disproportionate burden of social suffering (Adelson 2005; Dossa 2003, 2005), and their voices are often silenced. Aboriginal women remain under-represented or ignored in policy literature on Aboriginal peoples and often excluded in decision-making processes in their homes and communities (Canada 1996). While many matriarchal social structures represented many First Nations communities pre-contact, colonization, with its combined racism and sexism, served to denigrate and marginalize Aboriginal women.

Stout and Kipling note that insofar as academic endeavours have singularly focused on Aboriginal women's problems, they have "pathologized these women's agency and realities" (1998, 7) and overlooked the heterogeneity among Aboriginal women and the myriad of ways that they function as agents of change. Master narratives from liberal Western feminists that have historically tended to downplay the differences between women, generated, for example, through processes of colonization, are being resisted by Aboriginal women, who call for indigenous sovereignty, sustainability, and social justice (O'Neil, Elias, and Yassi 1998; Sterritt 2007).

We move now to a critique of multiculturalism – a concept that has also silenced Aboriginal voices and depoliticized the voices of immigrant men and women.

Critique of Dominant Discourses: Multiculturalism from a Post-Colonial Feminist Perspective

The discourse of multiculturalism within the Canadian state has often obscured social inequities underpinned by intersecting gendered, classed, and raced relations. Bannerji (2000) brings to our attention the ways in which the discourse of multiculturalism sidesteps existing ideological practices and relations of ruling – and presents diversity in neutral terms. In her critique of Charles Taylor's (1992) call for recognition of specific cultural identities, Bannerji argues that "what is necessary to deal with cultural contestation ... is not an accolade of worth, or a statement of their equal value, but rather a political organization, even constitutional reforms, which guarantee structural and legal conditions to all members of the society to wage struggles at many levels, including that of culture" (2000, 149). A PCF critique gets to the very roots of examining how inequities are reproduced – and sustained – through the relations of ruling and ideological formations that are overlooked in discourses of "cultural recognition." Intra-ethnic class relations and relations of ruling within the Canadian state are obscured by notions of culture that treat "ethnic" groups as homogeneous ("you have a common culture"), implying shared belief systems, when in fact, intra-ethnic heterogeneity is as prevalent within so-called ethnic groups as it is among the "Euro-Canadian" population. Crucial to any critique of multiculturalism is the striking absence of First Nations in the representation of who Canada is. We need to examine, more closely, how the Canadian state is sustained by class interests and intragroup exploitation, often a carry-over from legacies of colonial ideologies. The ideology of multiculturalism, which "celebrates" an "apoliticized diversity," falls short of disentangling the complex social relations that reproduce and sustain the ruling apparatus within the Canadian state.

Important to our implementation of PCF as a powerful analytic tool was the realization of the inadequacies of theoretical frameworks derived in Western European settings for conducting research with non-European communities. Some of the more salient PCF features foregrounded in our community research in Canada and India relate to recognizing intersectional oppressions; critical reflexivity regarding researcher privilege; concern for representation; accounting for vestiges of colonialism, including racialization and classism; recognizing shifting, hybrid identities for women; tracking the influence of history and place; and listening to silenced voices. We are struck by the analytic leverage represented by PCF. These analytic features have yielded new insights for us within the context of community research.

A Post-Colonial Feminist Critique of Community Research

In the application of PCF to community research, we have questioned the notion of *community*, in particular, problematizing (a) essentialist constructions of community, (b) researchers' claims to community partnerships, and (c) the historically grounded relations of power that can be inferred by *community*. As we have engaged in research with different ethnocultural groups, we have not assumed that people from the same ethnocultural group constitute a community. While deep cultural traditions and religious, social, personal, and political interests bring people together, groups are never homogeneous. Nor have we assumed that we could become part of "their community," even when ethnicity or professional identities were shared. We, therefore, view *community* as a fluid social construct that has political, social, religious, and cultural relevance at different points in time; community is not a static concept. This being said, for the purposes of conducting research, we recognize different social formations and their fluidity, and the processes of engagement that are central to the conduct of the research – for example, who to approach, how and when to approach people, understanding group norms, the processes of building alliances, balancing scientific integrity with advocacy, and the multitude of other factors that need to be understood as one embarks upon community-based research.

Essentialist and reductionist notions of community have been equally contested and dismissed by critical feminist scholars in India. As argued by

Sangari, "any single basis of 'community' will not only be ephemeral or provisional, liable to fragmentation by other cross-cutting affiliations, but it cannot represent the full spectrum of social divisions and locations, cultural diversities and aspirations" (1995, 3292). She further critiques, particularly in the context of enmeshing religious community and personal law in India, how community entities could be both punitive and protective to women but protective more on the basis of patriarchal assumptions. Sangari (1995) emphasizes the need to focus on multiple overlapping patriarchies and how that overlap calls into question the principle of demarcating communities. At the same time, *Dalit* ("lower" caste) feminists like Swathy Margaret argue that they have not much in common with the urban, educated, English-speaking feminists in India, as these upper-caste feminists do not have a "caste to be bothered about" (2005, 4). Margaret argues that "not all *Dalit* bodies are one, not all female bodies are one" (4) and notes, in the context of caste-gender dynamics, that while Dalit feminism has points of identification with both feminist and caste movements, it is important for Dalit feminism to retain its unique voice and carve out its own space through which it can both contribute to and benefit from these movements.

Post-colonial feminism supports such arguments against universalizing tendencies and meta-narratives and allows an analysis that takes into account the foundational differences among women that stem from various social stratifications like race, social class, caste, and sexuality and enables listening to multiple voices (Raju 2002). This is similar to what PCF scholar Mohanty (2003) writes about "feminism without borders," a feminism that acknowledges the differences, conflicts, and containment that borders represent, as opposed to a border-less feminism or universal sisterhood.

Khan, in her work with women living in the slums of Delhi, found such parallels of feminism without borders and the dynamic notions of community at play in the everyday lives of the slum women. Although women in slums generally interacted with and took help from their own caste groups, it was not unusual to observe women cutting across kin and caste group. In the study (Khan in press), which explored the socio-economic and cultural context of tuberculosis (TB) and the lived experiences of women patients, because of the social implications of TB, women faced serious difficulties in going every day to the TB centre for the intake of medicines, particularly when they were forced to hide their illness from their own families. In order not to arouse any suspicion, quite often they would visit the TB clinic on the pretext of going for groceries or fetching water from the local community tap, and they would have another woman (from the same or a different caste or religious group) accompany them in a way to defy the patriarchal forces of surveillance, power, and control. Feelings of solidarity and community arose from mutuality and the recognition of common problems and interests – often opposing essentialist notions of community.

A second matter brought into focus through a post-colonial feminist lens is that of partnerships for the sake of community research. Regardless of feminist values such as reciprocity and mutuality, for the most part in our research with communities, partnerships have had to be negotiated, and trust established. *This takes time,* and the time schedules of the community and the researcher are often different. Agendas need to be made explicit in the negotiation process. For example, in Anderson's research with women who had immigrated to Canada, some women participated out of altruism: they felt that this research may not be of benefit to them, but might help other women in the future. Some women also said that the researchers were the first people who had had the time to listen to their stories; they looked forward to "interviews" to engage in conversation about issues in their lives. With other research participants, contextual constraints influenced the research process. In Reimer-Kirkham's research with nurses, even though the nurses and academic researchers shared a common commitment and entered into a partnership to enhance patient care, the nurses were constrained by the clinical demands of their practice, leaving them with little time for research. It behoves the researcher to be cognizant of the context of nursing practice; negotiation is, therefore, an ongoing process.

Similarly, in Reimer-Kirkham's Partnering with Aboriginal Communities Project, partnership has been negotiated and renegotiated. Cargo et al. (2008) astutely observe that participation may be an ideal of community research on the part of academic researchers, but this ideal may, in fact, compete with indigenous peoples' rights to self-determination. Smith (1999) alerts us to the widespread ideal of research as benefiting "marginalized" or vulnerable communities, a notion that she locates in Western ideology. A further observation that Smith makes is that a focus on community assumes that the locus of the problem lies within the community itself, rather than with other social or structural issues. So, words such as *partnerships* and *community* must be used with caution in academic settings, lest we claim more than we can deliver.

Finally, the construct of *community* can, paradoxically, be inscribed with relations of power. For example, for Aboriginal peoples the concept of community is embedded in a (dis)connection to place and the "land," and typically, this connection is imbued in (neo)-colonial dominance. Smith traces the processes by which traditional Aboriginal territories were appropriated from indigenous cultures and then "gifted back" as reservations, "reserved pockets of land" (1999, 51). To refer to "Aboriginal communities" thus invokes colonized history and place, increasingly disconnected from the previous generations and traditions. Yet, for non-Aboriginal researchers, the notion of community is typically deemed a neutral descriptor, devoid of such ties to history and place. PCF and indigenous theorizing alert us to the multiple ways in which colonizing histories can be implicated in community research.

Our conversation and research exemplars have made evident the enriched analytic capacity of PCF theories, but as with all theoretical frameworks, we are also alert to some of the shortcomings of PCF theorizing, to which we now turn.

Problematizing Post-Colonialism

Post-colonialism is not without its critics, and we would be remiss if we did not address some of their issues. Scholars, such as Dirlik (1994, 2002), have drawn attention to post-coloniality's primary attentiveness to questions of cultural identity. Dirlik argues that this has disassociated "questions of culture and cultural identity from the structures of capitalism, shifting the grounds for discourse to the encounter between the colonizer and the colonized, unmediated by the structures of political economy within which questions of culture had been subsumed earlier" (2002, 432). A cogent argument that runs through this critique is the extent to which post-colonial discourse ignores the active colonialism of transnational corporatism. Miyoshi notes that "the current academic preoccupation with 'post-coloniality' and multiculturalism looks suspiciously like another alibi to conceal the actuality of global politics ... colonialism is even more active now in the form of transnational corporatism" (1993, 728). Colonizing processes, it is pointed out, are not in the past but remain central to ongoing discursive and social formations.

Post-colonialism has also been criticized in India, by scholars like Aijaz Ahmad. One of Ahmad's main contentions is about the *post* in *post-colonialism* and how that seems to indicate more a sense of euphoria (than a sense of loss) when there's not much reason for celebration, given the ongoing "creeping annexation of the globe for the dominance of capital over labouring humanity" (1997, 364). The other major criticism relates to how the term *post-colonial* gets applied so widely, "universally" throughout the globe, and its usage tends to include colonialism itself and often anything that comes after it, making *post-colonial* what Ahmad reads as something of "a remorseless universality" (366). However, despite this "universality" in usage, *post-colonial* remains limited to the theoretical work done by a select group of academic elites. This criticism of universality, and of the tendency "to appropriate the whole world as its raw material" and to ignore the issue of "historically sedimented differences" (370), is shared by other scholars such as feminist Kukum Sangari. In her early essay, "The Politics of the Possible," Sangari argues how, on the one hand, "the world contracts into the West," that is, a Eurocentric perspective is imposed on the cultural products of the Third World, while on the other hand, "the West expands into the World," as late capitalism muffles and homogenizes the world and all its cultural production (1987, 183). The arguments of these scholars coalesce around overcoming "aggrandizements of postcolonial theory" (Ahmad 1997, 369), regaining its more specific meaning, recognizing how the history of the West and non-West are "irrevocably different and irrevocably shared" (Sangari 1987, 185), and accounting for how each has shaped the other in specific ways.

Clearly, how the term *post-colonial* is understood in Canada and how it is understood in countries, such as India, that experienced colonial rule followed by the struggle for independence are quite different. Such differences are discernible particularly in observations of everyday life. For example, in travels to "past" colonial societies (such as India or the Caribbean), we have been struck by the language of "freedom" in everyday conversations. Phrases such as "after the end of 'foreign rule'" and "since we gained our freedom" signal a historical transition and the sense of nationhood brought to the lives of ordinary people. "Freedom" came at the time when the "colonial powers left." *Freedom at Midnight*, a book about the eclipse of the British Raj, documents the emergence of the new India (Collins and Lapierre 1975). However, this "freedom" did not mean an immediate end to the issues and challenges faced by the country. For example, Sumit Sarkar notes that the achievement of Indian independence in August 1947 witnessed the greatest transition, which in many ways remains grievously incomplete, and "many of the aspirations aroused in the course of the national struggle remained unfulfilled" (1985, 4). So, while it might be argued that "freedom," within the discourse of "past" colonized countries, does not mean an end to poverty, hardships, and gender and social inequalities or the fulfillment of people's hopes and aspirations, yet that demarcating timeline (when "freedom" was realized) holds significance in specific ways. Independence from "foreign rule" means a redefinition of self, from the "inferior," "subordinated," and colonized "Other," to a renewed sense of personhood and nationhood. In this sense, we use the term *post-colonial* to mean a new historical consciousness, underpinned by complex social processes within given geographical contexts. Many of us from colonized societies see a definite juncture between "before" and "after" independence from colonial powers. This is not to deny the continuing role of transnational corporatism. We are cognizant of ongoing neo-colonialism in societies that were colonized. The point to be stressed here, however, is the centrality of place in conceptualizations of post-colonialism. The concepts we have discussed have currency in Canada, but they may be best understood as decolonizing practices to address the ongoing experiences of Aboriginal peoples and peoples from past colonial societies, who are "Othered," marginalized, and racialized, as well as to highlight the ways in which different social formations are reproduced.

To conclude, we explore the intersection of theory, methodology, and methods in regard to post-colonial feminist and community-based research.

Concluding Comments: The Intersection of Theory, Methodology, and Methods

Our intent in this chapter was not only to explicate the epistemological and theoretical underpinnings of PCF scholarship, but more importantly, we wanted to shed light on how these concepts are taken up in different spaces and how they inform the research agenda, using, as examples, our research conducted in Canada and India. We argue that it is misleading to construct Canada as a "post-colonial nation" – Aboriginal peoples and peoples from past colonial nations who now make Canada home may not see colonizing practices as a thing of the past within the Canadian state (Battiste 1998; Battiste, Bell, and Findlay 2002; Bannerji 2000). We, therefore, need to distinguish between what we mean by *post-colonial nations* and doing PCF research. By calling our research post-colonial, we are not implying that Canada is post-colonial in the same way that countries such as India are post-colonial. Rather, a critique of the colonizing project informs our work. This critique, we believe, has relevance for community-based research in countries such as Canada.

While similar threads run throughout different kinds of critical feminist scholarship, concepts such as positionality in histories of colonization and power imbalances that are *historically* inscribed and socially reproduced have a firm footing in PCF epistemology, influencing methodological approaches and the interpretive lens brought to the analytic process. We

(Anderson 2002; Khan et al. 2007; Reimer-Kirkham and Anderson 2002) have articulated the essential elements of post-colonial research, underscoring the following: an analytic framework that allows for the examination of intersectionalities; connecting the micro and macro levels of analysis; bringing out the voices of those who have been silenced; and commitment to social change.

The methods used in post-colonial feminist inquiry, and the theoretical and methodological rigour demanded, bear similarity to other approaches to feminist inquiry. Neither qualitative nor quantitative methods are privileged; methods of data collection and analysis are used that are consistent with the questions asked. Measurement and statistical analyses that would, for example, illuminate income disparities among different groups, and how these disparities intersect with other variables, are as important as in-depth narratives and narrative analysis. Likewise, the complexities of interviewing and data analyses when different language groups are included are as germane to PCF research as they are in other approaches committed to the inclusion of diverse populations in research studies. What we emphasize in PCF *analytic processes* is writing in the subjugated voices and drawing upon theoretical perspectives that help us to make the connections between everyday experience and contexts and categories (such as race) that are historically inscribed and socially and politically reproduced through ongoing relations of power and colonizing processes. Concepts then, such as race, racialization, and culture, as they intersect with gender, social class, caste and other social relations are pivotal to the post-colonial and decolonizing analytic processes.

Given the social mandate of post-colonial feminist research, knowledge translation and engagement with policy makers to bring about social and political change is a key methodological component of community-based research projects. The methodology is set up to engage with policy makers from the very beginning. Research is viewed as an iterative process. Data collection and analysis are treated as concurrent processes with ongoing dialogue with policy makers; the questions that policy makers ask are integrated into the actual research questions. Again, we do not claim that this approach is unique to PCF research – rather, we argue that it is an important component of praxis-oriented research and that it is driven by the theoretical orientation that underpins such research.

Putting into practice a PCF perspective as we engage in community-based research draws attention to the embeddedness of past historical processes and present colonizing practices. While research from a PCF perspective is underpinned by methodological and ethical challenges similar to those of other critical feminist research, the aim of PCF scholarship is to encourage conversation among those with histories that are "irrevocably different and irrevocably shared" (Sangari 1987, 185) and, through this engagement, to disrupt dominant "master narratives." We believe that post-colonial feminist, black feminist, Aboriginal, and other critical feminist epistemologies can come together in an alliance around common issues situated in different histories to engage in discourse that will transcend the past and look towards new horizons of hope. The aim is to construct, in conjunction with existing paradigms, new paradigms of inquiry across the health sciences, social sciences, and the humanities that are inclusive of different ways of knowing and that have greater explanatory power than those we have known before.

NOTES

1 The term *immigrant woman of Colour,* widely used within the Canadian state, is not an uncontested category. We contend that it emphasizes the immigrant status of people who are not from dominant Euro-Canadian groups, and it reinscribes colonizing processes. So, while those of us from post-colonial societies may see Canada as "home," and think of ourselves as "Canadian," we may be perceived as being from "some place else" – underscored by the nuanced question, "Where are you from?" in contexts where such a question emphasizes our "Otherness."

2 The demographics of immigrant women entering Canada have changed. Many are now highly educated and fluent in English. Yet, their incomes lag well behind the incomes of Canadian-born women with equivalent education (Statistics Canada 2008).

3 We use the term *Third World* as it is used within Western nations to refer to societies that are economically disadvantaged (were colonized). However, we find the term *Countries of the South* more acceptable, as it positions us in relation to our geography rather than to a colonial past in which we continue to be constructed as "underdeveloped."

REFERENCES

Adelson, Naomi. 2005. "The Embodiment of Inequity: Health Disparities in Aboriginal Canada." *Canadian Journal of Public Health* 96(2): S45-S61.

Ahluwalia, Sanjam. 2003. "Rethinking Boundaries: Feminism and (Inter)nationalism in Early-Twentieth-Century India." *Journal of Women's History* 14(4): 188-95.

Ahmad, Aijaz. 1997. "Postcolonial Theory and the 'Post-' Condition." *Socialist Register* 33: 353-81.

Anderson, Joan M. 2002. "Toward a Postcolonial Feminist Methodology in Nursing Research: Exploring the Convergence of Postcolonial and Black Feminist Scholarship." *Nurse Researcher* 9(3): 7-27.

Anderson, Joan M., Connie Blue, and Annie Lau. 1991. "Women's Perspectives on Chronic Illness: Ethnicity, Ideology, and Restructuring of Life." *Social Science and Medicine* 33(2): 101-13.

Anzaldua, Gloria. 1987. *Borderlands/La Frontera*. San Francisco: Aunt Lute.

Bahri, Deepika. 2004. "Feminism in/and Postcolonialism." In N. Lazarus, ed., *The Cambridge Companion to Postcolonial Literary Studies*, 199-220. Cambridge: Cambridge University Press.

Bannerji, Himani. 2000. *The Dark Side of Nation: Essays on Multiculturalism, Nationalism and Gender*. Toronto: Canadian Scholars' Press.

Battiste, Marie. 1998. "Enabling the Autumn Seed: Toward a Decolonized Approach to Aboriginal Knowledge, Language and Education." *Canadian Journal of Native Education* 22(1): 16-27.

Battiste, Marie, Lynne Bell, and Len Findlay. 2002. "Decolonizing Education in Canadian Universities: An Interdisciplinary, International, Indigenous Research Project." *Canadian Journal of Native Education* 26(2): 82-95.

Bhabha, Homi. 1994. *The Location of Culture*. London: Routledge.

Brah, Avtar. 1996. *Cartographies of Diaspora: Contesting Identities*. London and New York: Routledge.

Brewer, Rose. 1993. "Theorizing Race, Class and Gender: The New Scholarship of Black Feminist Intellectuals and Black Women's Labour." In S.M. James and A.P.A. Busia, eds., *Theorizing Black Feminisms: The Visionary Pragmatism of Black Women*, 13-30. London: Routledge.

Browne, Annette. 2007. "Clinical Encounters between Nurses and First Nations Women in a Western Canadian Hospital." *Social Sciences and Medicine* 64: 2165-76.

Brydon, Diana. 2003. "Canada and Postcolonialism: Questions, Inventories, Future." In Laura Moss, ed., *Is Canada Postcolonial? Unsettling Canadian Literature*, 49-77. Waterloo, ON: Wilfrid Laurier University Press.

Canada. 1996. Royal Commission on Aboriginal Peoples. *Report of the Royal Commission on Aboriginal Peoples*. Vol. 3, *Gathering Strength*. Ottawa: Author.

Cargo, Margaret, Treena Delormier, Lucie Lévesque, Kahente Horn-Miller, Alex McComber, and Ann Macaulay. 2008. "Can the Democratic Ideal of Participatory Research Be Achieved? An Inside Look at an Academic-Indigenous Community Partnership." *Health Education Research* 23(5): 904-14.

Chakraborty, Dipesh. 1992. "Provincializing Europe: Postcoloniality and the Critique of History." *Cultural Studies* 6(3): 337-57.

Collins, Larry, and Dominique Lapierre. 1975. *Freedom at Midnight*. New York: Simon and Schuster.

Collins, Patricia Hill. 1990. *Black Feminist Thought: Knowledge, Consciousness, and the Politics of Empowerment*. Cambridge, MA: Unwin Hyman.

Dirlik, Arif. 1994. "The Postcolonial Aura: Third World Criticism in the Age of Global Capitalism." *Critical Inquiry* 20(2): 328-56.

–. 2002. "Rethinking Colonialism: Globalization, Postcolonialism and the Nation State." *Interventions* 4(3): 428-48.

Dossa, Parin. 2003. "The Body Remembers: A Migratory Tale of Social Suffering and Witnessing." *International Journal of Mental Health* 32(3): 50-73.

–. 2005. "'Witnessing' Social Suffering: Testimonial Narratives of Women from Afghanistan." *BC Studies* 147: 27-49.

Frankenberg, Ruth. 1993. *White Women, Race Matters: The Social Construction of Whiteness.* Minneapolis: University of Minnesota Press.

Gandhi, Leela. 1998. *Postcolonial Theory: A Critical Introduction.* New York: Columbia University Press.

Gedalof, Irene. 1999. *Against Purity: Rethinking Identity with Indian and Western Feminisms.* London: Routledge.

hooks, bell. 1984. *Feminist Theory: From Margin to Centre.* Cambridge, MA: South End Press.

Joseph, Cynthia. 2009. "Postcoloniality and Ethnography: Negotiating Gender, Ethnicity and Power." *Race Ethnicity and Education* 12(1): 11-25.

Khan, Koushambhi Basu. In press. "Understanding the Gender Aspects of Tuberculosis: A Narrative Analysis of the Lived Experiences of Women with TB in Slums of Delhi, India." *Health Care for Women International.*

Khan, Koushambhi Basu, Heather McDonald, Jennifer Baumbusch, Sheryl Reimer-Kirkham, Elsie Tan, and Joan M. Anderson. 2007. "Taking up Postcolonial Feminism in the Field: Working through a Method." *Women's Studies International Forum* 30: 228-42.

Lorde, Audre. 1984. *Sister Outsider.* Trumansburg, NY: Crossing Press.

Mani, Lata. 1987. "Contentious Traditions: The Debate on Sati in Colonial India." *Cultural Critique,* 7: 119-56.

–. 1990. "Multiple Mediations: Feminist Scholarship in the Age of Multinational Reception." *Feminist Review* 35: 24-41.

Margaret, Swathy M. 2005. "Dalit Feminism." Editorial. *Experience, Introspection and Expression* 1(7/8): 3-6. Magazine of the Ambedkar study circle.

McCall, Leslie. 2005. "The Complexity of Intersectionality." *Signs: Journal of Women in Culture and Society* 30(3): 1771-800.

Miyoshi, Masao. 1993. "A Borderless World? From Colonialism to Transnationalism and the Decline of the Nation-State." *Critical Inquiry* 19(4): 726-51.

Mohanty, Chandra Talpade. 2003. *Feminism without Borders: Decolonizing Theory, Practicing Solidarity.* Durham: Duke University Press.

Moss, Laura. 2003. *Is Canada Postcolonial? Unsettling Canadian Literature.* Waterloo, ON: Wilfrid Laurier University Press.

Narayan, Uma. 2000. "Essence of Culture and Sense of History: A Feminist Critique of Cultural Essentialism. In U. Narayan and S. Harding, eds., *Decentering the Center,* 80-100. Bloomington: Indiana University Press.

O'Neil, J., B. Elias, and A. Yassi. 1998. "Situating Resistance in Fields of Resistance: Aboriginal Women and Environmentalism." In M. Lock and P. Kaufert, eds., *Pragmatic Women and Body Politics,* 260-86. New York: Cambridge University Press.

Phoenix, Ann. 2009. "De-colonising Practices: Negotiating Narratives from Racialised and Gendered Experiences of Education." *Race, Ethnicity and Education* 12(1): 101-14.

Prakash, Gyan. 1992. "Postcolonial Criticism and Indian Historiography." *Social Text* 31/32: 8-19.

Raju, Saraswati. 2002. "We Are Different, But Can We Talk?" *Gender, Place and Culture* 9(2): 173-77.

Reimer-Kirkham, Sheryl. 1998. "Nurses' Experiences of Caring for Culturally Diverse Clients." *Clinical Nursing Research* 7(2): 125-46.

–. 2003. "The Politics of Belonging and Intercultural Health Care Provision." *Western Journal of Nursing Research* 25(7): 762-80.

Reimer-Kirkham, Sheryl, and Joan Anderson. 2002. "Postcolonial Nursing Scholarship: From Epistemology to Method." *Advances in Nursing Science* 25(1): 1-17.

Sangari, Kumkum. 1987. "The Politics of the Possible." *Cultural Critique* 7: 157-86.

–. 1995. "Politics of Diversity: Religious Communities and Multiple Patriarchies." *Economics and Political Weekly* 30(51): 3287-310.

Sarkar, Sumit. 1985. *Modern India, 1885-1947.* Delhi: Macmillan.

Smith, Linda Tuhiwai. 1999. *Decolonizing Methodologies: Research and Indigenous Peoples.* London: Zed Books.

Spivak, Gayatri Chakravorty. 1985. "The Rani of Sirmur: An Essay in Reading the Archives." *History and Theory* 24(3): 247-73.

–. 1988. "Can the Subaltern Speak?" In C. Nelson and L. Grossberg, eds., *Marxism and the Interpretation of Culture,* 271-313. London: Macmillan.

Statistics Canada. 2008. Catalogue no. 97-563-XWE2006002. Ottawa. Released May 1.

Sterritt, A. 2007. *Racialization of Poverty: Indigenous Women, the Indian Act and Systematic Oppression.* Report prepared for Vancouver Status of Women's Racialization of Poverty Project, Vancouver, BC. http://www.vsw.ca/Documents/IndigenousWomen_DEC2007FINAL.pdf.

Stout, Dion Madeleine, and Gregory D. Kipling. 1998. *Aboriginal Women in Canada: Strategic Research Directors for Policy Development.* Ottawa: Status of Women Canada.

Taylor, Charles. 1992. *Multiculturalism and the Politics of Recognition.* Princeton, NJ: Princeton University Press.

Trinh, T. Minh-Ha. 1989. *Woman, Native, Other: Writing Postcoloniality and Feminism.* Bloomington: Indiana University Press.

Vedeld, Trond, and Abhay Siddham. 2002. "Livelihoods and Collective Action in Slum Dwellers in a Mega-city (New Delhi)." Paper presented at The Commons in an Age of Globalisation, the Ninth Biennial Conference of the International Association for the Study of Common Property, Victoria Falls, Zimbabwe, 17-21 June.

Williams, Patrick, and Laura Chrisman, eds. 1994. *Colonial Discourse and Post-Colonial Theory: A Reader.* New York: Columbia University Press.

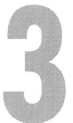

Feminist Demands, Dilemmas, and Dreams in Introducing Participatory Action Research in a Canada-Vietnam Capacity-Building Project

LEONORA C. ANGELES

Feminist academics and planners who incorporate participatory action research (PAR) principles in their community-based research and capacity-building work encounter many requirements (demands), challenges (dilemmas), and prospects (dreams) in their work. These demands, dilemmas, and dreams are magnified in complex international capacity-building programs that employ university-community partnerships. I explore why and how the incorporation of feminist PAR (FPAR) principles within university-community partnerships for both research-focused collaboration and capacity-building work could be difficult because of institutional and bureaucratic practices embedded within gendered hierarchical power relations and lines of authority, which influence the acceptability and attitudes towards FPAR and community-based research in universities. Here, I review the current literature on capacity building and feminist PAR or FPAR to find potential synergy in their principles. I analyze project documents and my own participant observation notes, as well as those taken by student interns, graduate students, and staff during workshops, meetings, study tours, and fieldwork in a Canada-Vietnam capacity-building program, called Localized Poverty Reduction in Vietnam (LPRV). I worked in the LPRV Program from 1998 to 2003 as a faculty research associate at the UBC Centre for Human Settlements, where the program is based. My tenure-track cross-appointment between the School of Community and Regional Planning and the Women's and Gender Studies Undergraduate Program

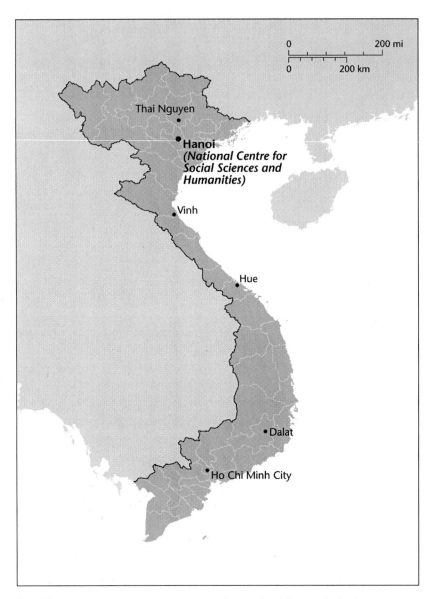

Figure 3.1   Vietnamese partner institutions in the Localized Poverty Reduction in
Vietnam (LPRV) project. The Canadian partner institutions are the University of British
Columbia's Centre for Human Settlements, the University of Laval's Department of
Geography, the Canadian International Development Agency, and the World University
Service of Canada.
Source: http://www.chs.ubc.ca/lprv/overviewF.html.

was made possible by the program, which needed expertise in gender analysis and participatory research approaches.

The place of PAR within university academic programs and international projects is discussed, using the case of LPRV as a capacity-building program in participatory project planning and policy assessment for poverty reduction. LPRV was funded by the Canadian International Development Agency (CIDA) and aimed to build the capacity of Vietnam academic institutions to assist local communities in meeting the challenges of reducing poverty. LPRV is based on the belief that universities have a role to play in sustainable poverty reduction by supporting democratic planning processes at the local level, and by integrating the research, teaching, and community work functions of universities. This objective connected with CIDA's poverty reduction strategy, and the Vietnamese government's National Program for Hunger Eradication and Poverty Reduction (HEPR), formulated in 1996 and officially inaugurated in 1999. LPRV program aims were partly shaped by the special features of Vietnam as a country in transition in its move towards a market economy, educational reforms, and integrated institutional linkages.

LPRV was initiated by academics from the University of British Columbia (UBC) and Vietnam's National Center for Social Science and Humanities (NCSSH) who had collaborated on a previous research capacity-building project called Social and Economic Impacts of *Doi Moi* (Renovation), funded by CIDA and by Canada's International Development Research Centre (IDRC) (Boothroyd and Pham Xuan Nam 2000).[1] Into the Localized Poverty Reduction in Vietnam program, UBC and NCSSH brought in Laval University and other Vietnamese university partners (some had previous working relationships with the proponents while a few had none) to involve other regional universities – Thai Nguyen University, Vinh University, Hue University, Dalat University, and Ho Chi Minh National University of the Social Sciences (see Figure 3.1). This well-funded international project on building capacity on project planning and policy assessment for localized poverty reduction appealed to the university administrators and local leaders in the fifteen target communes that were approached for initial discussions.

The programmatic focus on poverty reduction provided opportunities for Vietnamese and Canadian universities through LPRV to work together, using planning for commune-based poverty reduction projects as a means for developing capacity through learning by doing. The program's objective to adapt, test, and develop participatory methods and tools for project planning and policy assessment so that these tools could be brought back into the classrooms and continuing education programs (see Figure 3.2) led to commune-based projects such as micro-credit, micro-enterprise, water pump irrigation, health care, and livestock and poultry raising. The other objective of LPRV was to assist Vietnamese partner institutions in developing their human resources, library collections, and curricular offerings so that they could bring the program learning outcomes to students and work more effectively with local communities. The program also aimed to underscore the importance of PAR and other forms of participatory pedagogy and qualitative research that could help make universities more relevant to poverty reduction and community development work. The program thus provides a rich case to explore issues and challenges faced by FPAR practitioners involved in capacity building for both community-based research and curricular development in community-planning programs.[2]

Feminist Dreams, Capacity Building, and Participatory Action Research: Is Synergy Possible?

Globalization has affected universities around the world (Currie and Newson 1998), creating new forms of transnational cooperation between researchers in the North and in the South, such as collaborative university-community research partnerships and capacity-building programs, including FPAR, both locally and abroad (see Angeles and Boothroyd 2003; Schroeder 1997, 1998). Hence, there is a need to examine the common issues and themes in the literature on capacity building,[3] feminist PAR,[4] and university-community partnerships.[5] Although capacity building provides one of the foundations of realizing and sustaining feminist dreams to incorporate FPAR in academic and community settings, not all proponents of FPAR frame their work in terms of capacity building but, rather, appeal to gender equality, empowerment, or social justice objectives. By the time the LPRV was underway, there were already some concerns raised within and outside academic circles on the dangers and "dark side" of participation, particularly the type being pushed by international development agencies, as another form of social control to make the poor and marginalized more manageable (e.g., Cooke and Kothari 2001; Mosse 1994). Like development, social capital, empowerment, participation, and good governance, the term *capacity building* is a highly contested analytic concept (Angeles 2004), with the added burden of association with development management experts and international development agencies such as the World Bank and the United Nations Development Program (UNDP),[6] which have been pushing for "capacity development" as a new orientation in development aid. Those who embrace the term *capacity building,* or are aware of its limitations, often provide a protracted explanation of what capacities they are building, how, and for what purpose.

The term *capacity building,* however, has critical roots, as it reflects "fundamental discontent" with dominant approaches that focus on "the quantity rather than the quality of assistance and geared more to the internal agenda of the aid-giver than the recipient country's need to build capacity to plan and manage its own affairs" (Schacter 2000, 2-3). Capacity development, a macro-level change that encompasses micro- and meso-level capacity building, is envisioned to incorporate "the importance of stakeholders, participatory techniques, indigenous ownership, consensus and commitment" (Qualman and Bolger 1996, 2). Such a vision is able to address issues of voice, consensus, ownership, and participation, and thus makes capacity development (and by extension, capacity building) flexible enough to incorporate PAR and, by extension, FPAR principles of mutual learning and respect, reflexivity, reciprocity, responsiveness, responsibility, and intersectional analysis.

Although defined in various ways, and associated with different intellectual traditions, PAR is understood within LPRV to have some common elements:[7] (1) the participation in the research and ensuing action by community members as co-investigators; (2) the research exercise as an opportunity for consciousness raising and education of participants and facilitators; (3) the inclusion of popular, local, or indigenous knowledge, particularly that of the poor in general, poor women, ethnic minorities, and other disadvantaged groups; and (4) the inclusion of political action, participatory planning, and decision making (or "empowerment") based on a process of mutual learning and analysis, as well as continuous action and reflection (Chambers 1997; Fals-Borda and Rahman 1991; McTaggart 1997; Rahman 1993). As a form of qualitative research that addresses community problems and attempts to understand and change the world through the eyes of participants, it begins not with hypotheses to be proved or disproved, but with a flexible plan to explore a phenomenon or a community problem. The crux of PAR is the empowerment of disempowered groups and the search for practical approaches and methods to decentralize decision making, promoting democracy, diversity, and sustainability through community participation.[8] Thus, it was crucial for PAR participants in the Localized Poverty Reduction in Vietnam program to uncover and question stereotypes they may hold, particularly towards women, the poor, and ethnic minorities, and to discover unexpected knowledge or information, hidden by unchallenged assumptions and taken-for-granted "common sense" (Greenwood and Levin 1998).

Feminist PAR practitioners are clearly influenced by the above principles as they aim for the combination of research, activism, and social critique for the purpose of effecting social change and improved living conditions of marginalized groups. FPAR's emphasis has been on liberating oppressed groups through research as praxis, including the commitment to social change and progressive social movements, to honouring the lived experiences and knowledge of the people involved, and to paying attention to accountability, genuine collaboration, knowledge co-production, respect, reciprocity, and reflexivity in the research process (Gatenby and Humphries 1996, 2000; IFAD, ANGOC, and IIRR 2001; Penzhorn 2005). These feminist requirements in implementing PAR, however, are often lacking and remain challenging when undertaken in the context of community-based research and capacity-building projects involving international partnerships and university-community collaboration like LPRV.

Feminist Dilemmas: Introducing Feminist Participatory Action Research in Localized Poverty Reduction in Vietnam?

Although there are clear similarities between feminist research and participatory action research principles, there remain difficulties in introducing feminist principles in PAR-based capacity-building projects, particularly in post-socialist transition societies like Vietnam, with its own unique history of women's organizing and state–civil society relations. Perhaps a major source of these dilemmas is the lack of consensus on what feminism and PAR mean, and what happens when we combine feminist and PAR principles and practice. While the two share some similar principles and influences, they have also originated and grown independently of each other and are associated with various historical traditions, theories, philosophies, and ideological tendencies. So, what traditions and varieties of feminism or feminist theories or feminist movements (e.g., liberal, socialist, Marxist, radical, postmodern, neo-liberal, post-colonial, queer) are we talking about when we say "feminist research"? Conversely, what traditions of action research (e.g., traditional, radical, experiential, pedagogical) are we invoking when we say "participatory action research"? Do we necessarily connect feminist participatory action research with feminism as a form of political action, or feminist activism? Is feminist activism in itself a form of FPAR? Or should FPAR necessarily have a feminist activism component?

I raised these questions as I reflected on the possibilities and constraints in introducing FPAR in an international capacity-building project that has chosen gender equity, gender mainstreaming, and a gender analytic lens – not feminism nor feminist equality perspectives – as its framework in dealing with poverty issues and poverty-reduction measures. By the time LPRV was implemented in 1998, gender mainstreaming was already considered a globally accepted strategy to achieve gender equality by including gender perspectives and gender equality goals in research, advocacy, policy development, planning, implementation, resource allocation, and monitoring and evaluating projects and programs. Central to LPRV was the integration of gender analysis and ethnicity considerations as crosscutting themes in all its activities[9] – e.g., training workshops; network development; study tours; project planning, implementation, and evaluation; and curriculum development – in the universities and in work and operational arrangements in the communes.[10] Historically and intellectually, the original proponents of gender and development work and gender mainstreaming were clearly feminist in their orientation, given their political activist backgrounds. Over time, however, with their diffusion to many parts of the world and institutionalization in the mandates and commitments of development institutions, gender mainstreaming and gender analysis became part of another "technical fix" associated with and represented by "toolboxes" of approaches, frameworks, indicators, and checklists (Baden and Goetz 1997; Cornwall, Harrison, and Whitehead 2007), many of which were produced and used within LPRV.

The programmatic decision to deploy gender analysis and gender mainstreaming, instead of feminist analysis and feminist principles, was, on the one hand, both strategic and instrumentalist and, on the other hand, dilutive and apolitical. It was strategic and instrumentalist to use gender in order to render the LPRV gender team's arguments and activities palatable and meaningful to a skeptical (perhaps also anti-feminist) Vietnamese audience, and to increase the likelihood that they would be accepted and acted upon. To most LPRV women and men participants, composed of more than a hundred Canadian and Vietnamese academic faculty and students, as well as a group of at least thirty-five international student interns, and potentially thousands of Vietnamese community participants in its activities, feminism seemed to be a narrow and inappropriate framework, not to mention highly contested and contentious, with which to address its objectives in the Vietnamese context. Gender analysis seemed more inclusive, and its association with professional expertise in gender and development made it respectable and acceptable, rather than the radical-sounding feminist analysis. On the other hand, the decision also diluted the program's pro-woman and feminist social justice intentions (although these might exist only in the minds of key UBC, Laval, and NCCSH researchers) and rendered the gender team's arguments and activities rather apolitical and somewhat naive in their assumptions and expectations about how the deployment of gender could transform institutions and bureaucracies, especially universities. Perhaps this necessary depoliticization of gender was an inevitable outcome of the fact that LPRV had to operate within conservative institutions like universities and local governments, and work with academics in regional universities, many of whom have little or no background in political activism or feminist advocacy.

During many LPRV official events and public meetings, there was an observed self-censorship and "self-correction" among feminist LPRV participants, who avoided openly vocal criticisms and slippages into feminist language. They were diplomatic and highly conscious of not using the label "feminist" to qualify their research methods and planning processes, given the ideological and conceptual baggage of feminism in former colonies like Vietnam. But the more palatable focus on women's concerns and gender issues also provided openings for tackling real feminist "dilemmas and dreams," sans the label. I would also contend that the key women academic researchers from NCCSH, UBC, and Laval would no doubt identify with feminist principles and use feminist language within their small circle. To illustrate, shortly before the Definitions and Measurements of Poverty Workshop, in December 1998 in Ho Chi Minh City, Huguette Dagenais from Laval University facilitated a meeting of LPRV gender teams at the five universities to discuss issues and plan future program activities.[11] Dagenais emphasized that since gender pervades all aspects of life and thus of poverty, a gender lens should be applied to poverty-reduction work and their work in the program, noting that gender teams should not work in isolation but should be involved in all program decisions. A student intern summarizing the workshop proceedings noted:[12]

> Many women expressed their frustration that perhaps many of their ideas
> or comments were not taken seriously by their colleagues. Many felt they
> needed a deeper understanding of gender specifically and poverty reduc-
> tion generally to empower them in such situations. Some women felt that

they may be ostracized by their peers if they spoke out strongly on issues of gender. Many members are concerned with the information-sharing mechanisms in the project. Not all information is being passed down to all members and specifically to the gender teams.

Even then, the integration of gender analysis and sensitivity to ethnic minority issues, as well as participatory processes and other orientations that were considered new in the Vietnamese context, were met with some initial difficulties. Academic institutions, like other bureaucratic organizations, operate in gendered contexts, making the introduction of new orientations like gender, empowerment, and participatory approaches difficult within institutional settings (Angeles and Boothroyd 2003; Goetz 1997; Guijt and Shah 1998; Miller and Razavi 1998; Nelson and Wright 1995; Porter and Judd 2000; Savage and Witz 1992). This was due in part to the lack of common understanding of, or local vocabulary for, concepts such as gender, participation, good governance, social capital, learning by doing, or participatory action research – an understanding which in and by itself does not guarantee program success (Angeles and Gurstein 2000, 467). Both Vietnamese and Canadian participants in LPRV also had diverse understandings of these concepts, and differing attitudes towards various poverty reduction models and frameworks. Arriving at common understandings at the early stage in the project did not, of course, guarantee success in attaining program objectives, but this could have contributed to greater trust and team building among participants. There were also difficulties when the understandings of local cultures, power dynamics, and organizational capacities were rather limited and interpreted differently. The term *community*, for example, connotes cohesion and commonality of interests that may not be there (Guijt and Shah 1998, 8), especially when researchers are unaware of gendered contexts, local power differences, and new pressures faced by communities in light of transitional change.

Moreover, there was limited time in the Localized Poverty Reduction in Vietnam program for dialogue on cross-cultural differences and the transformative potentials of differences posed by language barriers and academic, political, and cultural traditions. Differences in incentives and reward structures between the Canadian and Vietnamese partners also affected the quality of transnational partnership. The Canadian team members, especially the senior ones, were most interested in pushing the program in the direction of mutually agreed upon terms of accountability (upward towards donor agencies, as well as downward towards commune residents) and addressing capacity-building needs. Junior Vietnamese and Canadian scholars on the teams were keen to see some good co-authored publications come out of the program, and appreciative of the research and travel per diem that largely went into savings and extra living expenses. Some Vietnamese participants also openly expressed interest in gaining skills from the program that would be valuable in seeking consulting positions with international agencies:

> While the Canadians may view the project as a vehicle for producing books and journal articles (like this one), most Vietnamese academics see international projects as an opportunity to augment their meagre salaries from the government. On both sides, the great demands placed on academic labour, that seems more elastic than ever before, also constrain the partners' ability to respond quickly to demands from the field, constant flow of communication, and frequency in face-to-face interactions between and among the Canadians and Vietnamese. (Angeles and Gurstein 2000, 469)

Lack of clear rewards and differing motivations in community-based research and development work were evident in how individual Vietnamese women and men in the LPRV program understood and negotiated their own place and share of the workload in the project.[13] Such negotiation and understanding were often expressed by participants informally and, normally, did not get space and voice in official meetings and discussions. A Canadian graduate student intern based at one of LPRV's partner universities explained such dynamics in one of his reports:[14]

> Mrs. Kim [not her real name] said that she found the proposed project very interesting, but expressed that it would be difficult for her to commit to it unless she received some kind of allowance, which I understand. She is currently building a new house, putting together proposals and applications for PhD scholarships, is a full-time teacher, and as she said, would have to pay a substitute if she were to be away from classes. Therefore, without more incentives other than interest and learning, I can imagine and understand how such work would not be high on her priorities ... However, she also said to me not to worry and that she would try to help me in "my project," which is very kind but sort of defeats the purpose.

Women academics were very active in the LPRV Program, despite time and resource constraints. Their academic and reproductive labour were stretched to the limits, as they too experienced gendered patterns of gendered inclusion and exclusion, similar to what are encountered by their counterparts in Western institutions of higher learning (e.g., Prentice and Stalker 1998). The original all-women LPRV gender team was later expanded to include men because of valid concerns over the program's conflation of "gender" and "women," and interpretation of gender issues as exclusively women's issues.[15] Vietnamese women in the LPRV program have expressed discomfort with the exclusion of men from gender team activities and have, in fact, welcomed and even pushed for the inclusion of men on the gender team and discussions of men and male identities in LPRV gender workshops.[16] The clamour from women to include men in gender discussions arose from a culturally derived understanding of gender relations in terms of sex-role complementarity, the importance of the family more than individuals, the acceptance of women's and men's comparative advantages, and the sexual division of labour, issues that are not necessarily equated with gender-based inequality and injustice.[17] The majority of participants also recognized that reorienting "male bias" (especially of key decision makers) could be a more effective strategy than direct confrontation. Gender and poverty concerns, to Vietnamese participants, did not mean problematizing men in terms of polarizing, oppositional, and dualist discourses on "women as victim, men as problem." Hence, in their fieldwork, the LPRV program's faculty and staff considered gender to be an important social variable, recognized that women face harsher obstacles, and took into account gendered poverty experiences based on position in the life cycle and the diversity of women and men among the poor and ethnic minorities.

Feminist Demand: Who Initiates Participatory Action Research?

Part of the dilemma in introducing FPAR has to do with the question of who initiates PAR, cognizant of a feminist demand for reflexivity, not just in the research process, but also in the relationship between the researchers and the researched in the community. Community-based PAR programs may have different initiators (community insiders or professional outsiders) and modalities of action (as shown in Figure 3.2) which affect their conduct and outcomes. When community insiders who have long lived in the area initiate PAR (Case A), there are generally fewer problems that arise in terms of language or communication, understanding of local culture and institutions, and trust building. Outsider-experts, who communicate the benefits of PAR to a community, may choose to either have only intermittent involvement while remaining detached (Case B) or make the commitment to

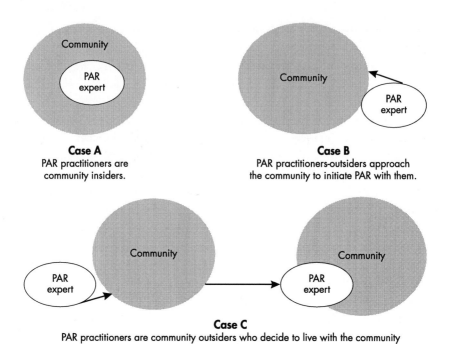

Case A
PAR practitioners are
community insiders.

Case B
PAR practitioners-outsiders approach
the community to initiate PAR with them.

Case C
PAR practitioners are community outsiders who decide to live with the community
during and beyond the PAR process, but still remain outsiders.

Figure 3.2   Initiators and modalities of participatory action research (PAR).
Source: L.C. Angeles, PLAN 548H - Participatory Planning Methods and Tools, School of
Community and Regional Planning, University of British Columbia.

live and work within the community permanently or semi-permanently
(Case C). In Case B, problems around commitment, time, and team building
often arise, while in Case C, these problems may easily diminish when the
erstwhile outsiders come to be accepted by the community. The challenge,
therefore, for both Cases B and C is to ensure that local people can learn and
assimilate PAR principles and methods so that such skills remain in the
community long after the outsiders are gone, or in other words, how to
move closer to Case A.

One may interpret LPRV program goals as consistent with a PAR program, although LPRV team members saw PAR only as part of their methods. Framing LPRV's commune projects as a form of PAR may be difficult,
given that the commune projects were not instigated by community members themselves but by academic-outsiders aiming for consensus building,
making LPRV closer to Case B than Case C.[18] LPRV could have effectively

combined Case A and Case B by relying on a small but growing number of Vietnamese staff in non-governmental organizations (NGOs) and academics, who are already well versed in the use of participatory development approaches, but this in itself could not address operational problems.[19]

The use of the terms *insider* and *outsider*, however, should not detract us from examining complex intracommunal differences and varying levels of participation among local people, especially women, who are all lumped together as "insiders," even though some of them face exclusions and vulnerabilities (Guijt and Shah 1998, 9-10). Successful PAR programs are said to require *consensus* among all stakeholders regarding the nature of PAR and the appropriate research agenda for transnational partnership (Schroeder 1997). Likewise, democratic community planning appropriate for the Vietnamese context had been understood within LPRV as a method of getting different stakeholders' inputs in meetings (i.e., getting to "D," using LPRV lingo) between the circles of academics, government officials, and poor members of the community (see Figure 3.3). However, this point of interaction "D" may ignore diversity within governments, communities, and academies and tend to reinforce the idea that simply bringing people together to engage in needs assessment or decision-making processes could lead to empowerment:

> If power is essentially about the "transformative capacity" of people or groups, then empowerment involves increasing people's capacity to transform their lives ... Offering the marginalized opportunities for consultation, without following this through with analysis about causes of oppression and feasible action to redress the causes, is unlikely to be empowering. For a process to be empowering, it also requires the development of iterative sequences that emphasize different discussions and skills at different points in time. To integrate other skills such as group organization, conflict resolution, management, and small enterprise development requires appropriate support and institutional flexibility. The lack of resources needed for such follow-up has led some to comment on the disempowering nature of participation. (Guijt and Shah 1998, 11)

Such visions of empowerment were difficult to achieve within LPRV because of limited project time and resources to create integrated and long-term support and engagement between international partners and Vietnamese institutions. Moreover, there remains some institutional devaluation of participatory development approaches in both Vietnamese and

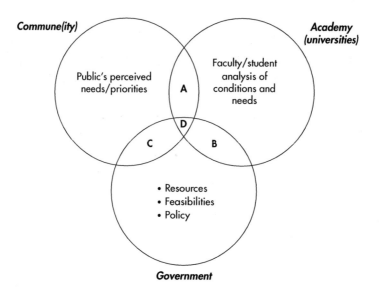

Figure 3.3 Getting to "D": Unifying concept that emerged from years one to three. *Source:* http://www.chs.ubc.ca/lprv/overviewF.html.

Canadian university settings. The diverse disciplinary backgrounds of Vietnamese academics influenced by their disciplinary perspectives and methodologies in the natural sciences, physics, and engineering affected their esteem and evaluation of the merits of PAR and feminist research methodologies. The interdisciplinary composition of LPRV teams reflected the reality that local community issues do not fit within narrow academic specializations and thus require multidisciplinary perspectives and skills in local planning (Boothroyd 1991). However, university academics generally preferred quantitative research methods that adhered to accepted standards (e.g., objectivity, reliability, and lack of bias), and some viewed qualitative research to be problematic, too anecdotal, and lacking in rigour and ability to make generalizations and predictions.[20] University-community collaboration thus clashes with an academic culture that tends to be highly structured, clearly defined, hierarchical, time limited, and obsessed with the use of scientific methods. In contrast, community engagement in the integrated nature of real life problems requires a mode of work that is highly flexible, adaptable, cooperative, and not limited to specific time frames but rather to satisfactory achievement of common objectives and goals (Dewar and Issac 1998).

Conclusion: What Feminism(s) Are We Bringing in Community-Based Action Research?

There are many openings for potential synergy between capacity-building programs involving international partnerships and feminist PAR. Principles that should guide community-university partnerships – clarity for the reasons and terms of partnership; common definition of problems; attention to the use of language; mutual trust, respect, and equality in relationships; flexibility and focus on processes; regular, ongoing assessments; and new ways of combining research, teaching, and social learning, especially in the curriculum (Holland 1999; Wilson and Whitmore 1995) – are also the principles that govern PAR and feminist research and teaching. Thus, international capacity-building programs are more likely to succeed in integrating FPAR principles when partners on both sides understand the common grounds and terms of their partnership for continued trust to be nurtured and for the process of mutual learning and empowerment to take place.

From my perspective, the LPRV program had been successful in building trust and developing mechanisms for mutual learning, and empowering program and community participants to the extent that it is possible to do so, given the constraints discussed above. The LPRV program strategically planned for the academic and non-academic outputs and results that would appeal to Vietnamese and Canadian university scholars and community development practitioners. Vietnamese scholars were given further support in doing research and writing for varied local, national, and international audiences, initially through co-authored or team-written publications, as had happened in the LPRV program and the first UBC-NCCSH project with CIDA (see Boothroyd and Pham Xuan Nam 2000). Using complementary funding from IDRC, support was given to networking among established and young Vietnamese scholars who were beginning to integrate feminist perspectives and gender analysis and combine quantitative and qualitative research traditions and data collection techniques. By invoking gender analysis and gender mainstreaming, LPRV invoked a depoliticized form of "feminism," limited in its transformative potential, but effective in creating openings for the demonstration and promotion of women's leadership, academic expertise, and other capacities, as well as gender-balanced representation in all activities.

Empowerment played out in the LPRV program mainly in terms of providing local autonomy in decision making. The LPRV program was also remarkable in giving greater autonomy to the Vietnamese partners in managing their financial resources and in determining their research focus, choice of communes, and the composition of their research team. Such adherence to participatory and democratic decision making in program administration and the allocation of resources is perhaps LPRV's best achievement in trying to practise "empowerment" and the democratic planning principles that it espouses within the universities and communes. Another achievement is its creation of time and space and allocation of resources for women academics in Vietnam to articulate and represent their problems and interests.

Feminist PAR practitioners may find donor-driven international development and capacity-building projects like the LPRV program to be flawed and inadequate, as they often fail to satisfy their feminist visions and requirements of being community driven and propelled by local issues and problems. In such a context, there are numerous challenges posed by *issues of inclusion and exclusion* arising from diversity, difference, and power imbalances between and within universities and community partners. FPAR practitioners often point to the need to deal with the negotiation of power relations and the transformative role of differences and historical reckoning in the action component and research process. In the end, the LPRV program's main weaknesses are perhaps its near-mythical relocation of a potentially transformative project (i.e., promoting participatory, bottom-up capacity building that integrates grassroots and gender-balanced participation) to inherently conservative non-transformative contexts (i.e., universities and local governments), using inherently bureaucratic resources and rules of the game (i.e., donor-drive development aid), and its unrealistic, if not naive, expectation that such relocation could produce transformative results.

The lessons learned from the potentials and constraints in integrating PAR and FPAR in international development work such as the LPRV program could contribute to shaping a new development research agenda and influence current thinking within academic institutions and the donor community. These could help foster new feminist models of collaborative research that involve not only North-South but also South-South partnerships to support research programs that are responsive to local needs and to national and/or sub-regional policy initiatives in developing countries like Vietnam. This could be done by a more pro-active and well-planned strategy in communicating their lessons to a wider audience that includes university students, faculty, and administrators, and NGOs working with grassroots organizations, academics, and funding agencies, as well as international donor agencies. More than ever, there is a great need for new forms of international cooperation and locally derived forms of feminist participatory action research to improve current practices, so that mistakes of the past do not bog us down or get resurrected in even more insidious forms.

NOTES

1 The UBC academics were Peter Boothroyd, Terry McGee, and Geoffrey Hainsworth. The key NCCHS senior academic researchers were Pham Xuan Nam, Do Thi Binh, Tran Thi Van Anh, Vu Tuan Anh, and Tran Trinh Luan, assisted by administrator Dang Anh Phuong. They were the key people involved in both LPRV and the Socio-economic Impacts of Doi Moi research project.

2 Although Vietnamese universities conduct LPRV-related work in different ways, these differences are reserved for another discussion to make some meaningful generalizations about the place of PAR within international capacity-development projects.

3 The formidable task of capacity building has already been explored in many studies (e.g., Grindle 1997; Gubbels and Koss 2000; Maconick and Morgan 1999; Morgan 1997, 1999; Schacter 2000).

4 See the following studies on the challenges of PAR in international contexts: Burkey (1993), Fals-Borda and Rahman (1991), McTaggart (1997), Nelson and Wright (1995), and Rahman (1993). Feminist action research as a methodology in local and international collaboration has been explored in Bowes (1996), Maguire (1987), and Slocum et al. (1995), Gatenby and Humphries (1996, 2000), Porter and Judd (2000), Miller and Razavi (1998).

5 For studies on partnerships in general, see Saxby (1999). On community-university partnerships, see Dewar and Issac (1998), and Zlotkowski (1998).

6 The UNDP defines *capacity building* as "the process by which individuals, organizations, institutions and societies develop abilities (individually and collectively) to perform functions, solve problems and set and achieve objectives" (UNDP 1997, 3). CIDA and other agencies that make up the Development Assistance Committee (DAC) of the Overseas Economic Cooperation for Development (OECD), the umbrella group of the richest donor countries, have also adopted capacity development in their programs.

7 This collective understanding, although uneven and not systematically captured or evaluated, emerged during various workshops and seminars from August 1998 to May 2003.

8 See website of the Participation Group of the Institute of Development Studies, University of Sussex, at http://www.ids.ac.uk.

9 Given space limitations and the complexity of gender and ethnicity issues within LPRV, these issues could not be discussed in this chapter.

10 Detailed discussion of LPRV activities and accomplishments could not be discussed here. For more information, see the LPRV website at http://www.chs.ubc.ca/lprv.

11 The gender team participants at this workshop included Do Thi Binh and Dang Anh Phuong from the NCSSH in Hanoi; Truong Thi Kim Chuyen and Tran Thi Kim Xuyen from the College of Social Sciences and Humanities in HCMC; Vu Thi Tung Hoa from Thai Nguyen University; Huynh Minh Phuong from Dalat University; Bui

Thi Tan from Hue University; Nguyen My Trinh from Vinh University; and Steffanie
Scott from the University of British Columbia.
12 Amy Gilchrist, writer for the LPRV newsletter, January 1999.
13 Field Notes, LPRV International Meeting, Ho Chi Minh City, December 1999.
14 Report by Jason Morris, CIDA intern for LPRV, dated 4-9 October 1999.
15 The first collaborative project funded by CIDA-IDRC had involved both women and
    men researchers, and it incorporated gender issues in the study of the household
    economy. See Part III of Boothroyd and Pham Xuan Nam (2000).
16 Field Notes, "Foundational Concepts, Methods and Tools in Poverty Reduction,"
    Local Workshops, Thai Nguyen and Vinh Universities, November 1998.
17 Field Notes, "Foundational Concepts, Methods and Tools in Poverty Reduction,"
    Local Workshops, Hue, Dalat, and Ho Chi Minh National Universities, December
    1998.
18 Except for graduate student interns, who had lengthier stays, there were no Canadian
    full-time project staff or faculty members who stayed in Vietnam for a period longer
    than two months.
19 The participation of non-governmental organizations (NGOs) in LPRV has been an
    issue, given the constricted space for NGO work in Vietnam, the reputation of
    NGOs among university academics, and funding guidelines in the project.
20 Field Notes, "Foundational Concepts, Methods and Tools in Poverty Reduction,"
    Local Workshop, Vinh University, November 1998.

REFERENCES

Angeles, Leonora. 2004. "New Issues, New Perspectives: Implications for Inter-
    national Development Studies." *Canadian Journal of Development Studies,*
    special issue on White Paper on International Development Studies, ed. Paul
    Bowles, 25 (1): 61-80.
Angeles, Leonora, and Peter Boothroyd. 2003. "Canadian Universities and Inter-
    national Development: Learning from Experience." In P. Boothroyd and L.
    Angeles, eds., special issue on Canadian Universities and International
    Development, *Canadian Journal of Development Studies* 24(2): 9-26.
Angeles, Leonora, and Penny Gurstein. 2000. "Planning for Participatory Capacity
    Development: The Challenges of Participation and North-South Partnerships
    in Capacity-Building Projects." *Canadian Journal of Development Studies* 21:
    447-78.
Baden, Sally, and Anne Goetz. 1997. "Who Needs [Sex] When You Can Have
    [Gender]?" In Kathleen Staudt, ed., *Women, International Development and
    Politics: The Bureaucratic Mire,* 18-36. Philadelphia: Temple University Press.
Boothroyd, Peter. 1991. "Developing Community Planning Skills: Applications of a
    Seven-Step Model." *CHS Research Bulletin.* Vancouver: University of British
    Columbia, Centre for Human Settlements.
Boothroyd, Peter, and Pham Xuan Nam. 2000. *Socioeconomic Renovation in
    Vietnam: The Origin, Evolution, and Impact of Doi Moi.* Ottawa: International
    Development Research Council.

Bringle, Richard Games, and Edward A. Malloy, eds. 1999. *Colleges and Universities as Citizens.* Needham Heights, MA: Allyn and Bacon.

Burkey, Stan. 1993. *People First: A Guide to Self-Reliant Participatory Rural Development.* London: Zed Books.

Chambers, Robert. 1997. *Whose Reality Counts? Putting the First Last.* London: Intermediate Technology Publications.

Cooke, Bill, and Uma Kothari. 2001. *Participation: The New Tyranny?* London and New York: Zed Books.

Cornwall, Andrea, Elizabeth Harrison, and Ann Whitehead, eds. 2007. *Feminisms in Development: Contradictions, Contestations and Challenges.* New York: Zed Books.

Currie, Jan, and Janice Newson, eds. 1998. *Universities and Globalization.* London: Sage.

Dewar, Margaret E., and Claudia B. Issac. 1998. "Learning from Difference: The Potentially Transforming Experience of Community-University Collaboration." *Journal of Planning Education and Research* 17: 334-47.

Fals-Borda, Orlando, and Muhammad Anisur Rahman, eds. 1991. *Action and Knowledge: Breaking the Monopoly with Participatory Action Research.* New York/London: Apex Press/Intermediate Technology Publications.

Gatenby, Bev, and Maria Humphries. 1996. "Feminist Commitments in Organizational Communication: Participatory Action Research as Feminist Praxis." *Australian Journal of Communication* 23(2): 73-88.

–. 2000. "Feminist Participatory Action Research: Methodological and Ethical Issues." *Women's Studies International Forum* 23(1): 89-105.

Goetz, Anne Marie, ed. 1997. *Getting Institutions Right for Women in Development.* London: Zed Books.

Greenwood, Davydd J., and Morten Levin. 1998. *Introduction to Action Research: Social Research for Social Change.* Thousand Oaks, CA: Sage.

Grindle, Merilee S., ed. 1997. *Getting Good Government: Capacity Building in the Public Sectors of Developing Countries.* Cambridge, MA: Harvard Institute for International Development.

Gubbels, Peter, and Catheryn Koss. 2000. *From the Roots Up: Strengthening Organizational Capacity through Guided Self-Assessment.* Oklahoma City: World Neighbors.

Guijt, Irene, and Meera Kaul Shah, eds. 1998.*The Myth of Community: Gender Issues in Participatory Development.* London: Intermediate Technology Publications.

Holland, Barbara A. 1999. "From Murky to Meaningful: The Role of Mission in Institutional Change." In Robert G. Bringle, Richard Games, and Edward A. Malloy, eds., *Colleges and Universities as Citizens,* 48-73. Needham Heights, MA: Allyn and Bacon.

IFAD, ANGOC, and IIRR, ed. 2001. *Enhancing Ownership and Sustainability: A Resource Book on Participation.* New Delhi/Manila: International Fund for Agricultural Development (IFAD), Asian NGO Coalition for Agrarian Reform and Rural Development (ANGOC), and International Institute of Rural Reconstruction (IIRR).

Maconick, Roger, and Peter Morgan, eds. 1999. *Capacity-Building Supported by the United Nations: Some Evaluations and Some Lessons.* New York: United Nations.

Maguire, Patricia. 1987. *Doing Participatory Research: A Feminist Approach.* Boston: Center for International Education, School of Education, University of Massachusetts.

McTaggart, Robin, ed. 1997. *Participatory Action Research: International Contexts and Consequences.* Albany: State University of New York Press.

Miller, Carol, and Shahra Razavi, eds. 1998. *Missionaries and Mandarins: Feminist Engagements with Development Institutions.* London: Intermediate Technology Publications.

Morgan, Peter. 1997. "The Design and Use of Capacity Development Indicators." Paper prepared for the Policy Branch of CIDA, December. http://www.mekonginfo.org/HDP/Lib.nsf/0/18A3C57E35F91A9E47256D80002F7C81/$FILE/CIDA%20-%20Capacity%20Development%20Indicators%201997.PDF.

–. 1999. "An Update on the Performance Monitoring of Capacity Development Programs." Paper presented at the Meeting of the Development Assistance Committee (DAC) Informal Network on Institutional and Capacity Development, Ottawa, 3-5 May 1999.

Mosse, David. 1994. "Authority, Gender and Knowledge: Theoretical Reflections on the Practice of Participatory Rural Appraisal." *Development and Change* 25: 497-526.

Nelson, Nici, and Susan Wright, eds. 1995. *Power and Participatory Development: Theory and Practice.* London: Intermediate Technology Publications.

Patton, Tracey Owens. 1999. "Ethnicity and Gender: An Examination of Its Impact on Instructor Credibility in the University Classroom." *Howard Journal of Communications* 10(2): 123-44.

Penzhorn, Cecilia. 2005. "Participatory Research: Opportunities and Challenges for Women in South Africa." *Women's Studies International Forum* 28: 343-54.

Porter, Marilyn, and Ellen Judd. 2000. *Feminists Doing Development: A Practical Critique.* Halifax/London: Fernwood/Zed Books.

Prentice, Susan, and Jacqueline Stalker. 1998. *The Illusion of Inclusion: Women in Post-Secondary Education.* Halifax: Fernwood.

Qualman, A., and J. Bolger. 1996. "Capacity Development: A Holistic Approach to Sustainable Development." CIDA website: http://www.acdi-cida.gc.ca/xpress/dex9608, downloaded 15 February 1999.

Rahman, Anisur. 1993. *People's Self-Development: Perspectives of Participatory Action Research: A Journey through Experience.* London: Zed Books.

Savage, Michael, and Anne Witz. 1992. *Gender and Bureaucracy.* Oxford: Blackwell.

Saxby, John. 1999. "Partnership in Question." An issues paper prepared for discussion at Setting the Stage for Tomorrow's Partnerships, International Cooperation Day, Ottawa, ON, 16-17 November 1999.

Schacter, Mark. 2000. *Capacity Building: A New Way of Doing Business for Development Assistance Organizations.* Policy Brief 6. Ottawa: Institute on Governance.

Schroeder, Kent. 1997. "Participatory Action Research in a Traditional Academic Setting: Lessons from the Canada-Asia Partnership." *Convergence* 30(4): 41-48.

–. 1998. *Pursuing Participatory Development through Cross-Cultural University Partnering: The Canada-Asia Partnership Experience.* Calgary, AB: Division of International Development, University of Calgary.

Slocum, Rachel, Lori Wichhart, Dianne Rocheleau, and Barbara Thomas-Slayter. 1995. *Power, Process and Participation – Tools for Change.* London: Intermediate Technology Publications.

UNDP. 1997. *Capacity Development.* Technical Advisory Paper 2. New York: United Nations Development Program. Cited in Schacter (2000, 2).

Wilson, Maureen G., and Elizabeth Whitmore. 1995. "Accompanying the Process: Principles for International Development Practice." *Canadian Journal of Development Studies* 16: 61-77.

Zlotkowski, Edward, ed. 1998. *Successful Service-Learning Programs: New Models of Excellence in Higher Education.* Bolton, MA: Anker.

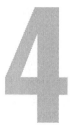

Travels with Feminist Community-Based Research
Reflections on Social Location, Class Relations, and Negotiating Reciprocity

SHAUNA BUTTERWICK

Between 1998 and 2004, I connected with a small group of women on low income in the lower mainland of Vancouver as they engaged with advocacy efforts to challenge repressive welfare policy and as they shifted their focus to experimenting with income-generating projects. While my initial entry was as an ally, we negotiated an agreement whereby my role expanded to include that of researcher. As an academic with a research grant, I was able to bring some resources (identified by them) to support their efforts. In exchange, I had an opportunity to participate in and document their discussions and their processes of learning. As a result, I learned about their everyday lived experiences of a repressive welfare system and "the ways in which a society reproduces itself and the powerful implications when certain groups become routinely excluded" (Carragata 2003, 572). Furthermore, I also became acquainted with these women's critical analysis of the system and their resistance to it, and the richness of their informal learning processes.

In this chapter, I focus on how this project offered a unique opportunity to explore some unexpected ways to work towards reciprocity, a fundamental concern in feminist community-based research (FCBR). Patti Lather defines reciprocity as "give and take, a mutual negotiation of meaning and power" (1991, 57). Lather calls for feminist researchers to work towards a maximalist approach, one that does not stop at engaging reciprocally for the sake of gathering rich data, but works dialogically: "central to establishing [reciprocity] is a dialogic research design where respondents are actively involved in the construction and validation of meaning" (63). In this narrative, I explore how class relations, among others, significantly shaped this project and my efforts at reciprocity, in complex and sometimes paradoxical ways. As Nesbit (2005, 7) argues: "Class still exists. As in Marx's time, all social life continues to be marked by the struggles and conflicts over access to the generation and distribution of wealth and status."

I hope this narrative sheds light on these challenges, paradoxes, and opportunities and that it contributes to an appreciation for the complexities of university-community partnerships, which are receiving much more attention now. In discussions about the "Third Mission" of universities, there is welcome recognition of the responsibility of universities *to* non-academic communities, but little commentary on social class and other forms of difference such as gender and race that profoundly shape social relations. Furthermore, there has been less attention given to what universities can learn *from* communities and how the resources that communities want, and the interests and perspectives they have, can challenge universities' traditional perspectives and ways of operating. Community-university engagements are not simple or quickly completed "outreach" projects; there must be recognition of the time needed to build mutually respectful engagements and the complex power relations that shape these relationships. Community is also a ubiquitous concept, and its multiple meanings are often not explored, nor is the assumption that communities are homogeneous. Communities are sites of struggle and contention, as much as they are places of solidarity. This "confessional tale" offers one account of a community-university engagement project, bringing a critical, feminist, and relational orientation to the discussion.

I offer this autobiographical account with caution. As Linda Alcoff (1991) so clearly outlines, power is always operating in these discursive spaces of representation of both self and others. Alcoff also points to how "whether I am speaking for myself or for others ... this representation is never a simple act of discovery" (10). My subjective experience of this project was far from a unified and coherent journey, although this retrospective analysis illuminates for me some threads and consistencies. I attempt to show these threads in the first part of the chapter, by describing how the project came into being, going into some detail about the pathways and network of relations that led to this connection. This is mapped out to illustrate a process of trial and error and serendipitous encounters, rather than any predetermined design. In the latter half of this discussion, I consider this account in light of the conceptualizations generated by feminist scholars whose work has significantly deepened my understanding of feminist community-based research, social relations, and reciprocity.

An Emergent Project

In the Beginning ...

While the FCBR project I recount here began in 1998, the pathways leading to this project were being developed many years earlier. My interest in women's learning was cemented during my nursing education and further expanded when I worked as a hospital and community-based nurse. I also learned a great deal about the importance of and the barriers to building mutually beneficial relationships between institutions and the communities being served by those organizations. These same issues continued to be of interest when I worked at a women's centre and subsequently began my graduate studies in adult education. During my graduate studies, I became active in several feminist organizations. These groups were challenging government policies that affected women, conducting community-based research, and advocating for change. My desire to shed light on women's learning, to work closely with women's communities, and to conduct participatory-oriented research continued with my academic position.

I met the women in this project when I was contracted by a joint federal and provincial committee to prepare a summary of evaluation studies of welfare-to-work programs, pointing to the effective components for lone mothers on assistance. Wanting to expand the information to include the perspective of single mothers, with the help of an anti-poverty organization, I held a focus group with twelve single mothers receiving social assistance. They readily offered their thoughts and experiences on what works and what doesn't work. The final report (Butterwick, Bonson, and Rogers 1998) included their ideas as well as the review of the evaluation studies. It was sent to the focus group participants and to the anti-poverty organization that helped host the focus group. I also submitted it to the government committee; however, my standpoint and conclusions did not fit well with the neo-liberal welfare reforms underway.

Not long after the report was finished, I was contacted by one of the women who had been part of the focus group. She invited me to a meeting in her home – an apartment in a social-housing complex, where the majority of residents were either receiving income assistance (IA) or were on low income. There were seven women at the meeting, all keen to organize against punitive welfare regulations and to work together to improve the opportunities for single mothers receiving IA. I joined that group, initially not with a specific request to conduct research, but as an expression of solidarity with their efforts and a way to exercise reciprocity for the time women had given to my evaluation project.

I was acutely aware of my middle-class privileged social location and raised it with the group, noting that I had never been poor, and for most of my life had lived a comfortable middle-class existence. I also had no children. This sparked a comment by one woman, who indicated that she too had, at one point, lived a middle-class life, but when the business she owned with her husband had failed and he left her, she experienced a downward spiral into poverty. I was reminded then, and on many other occasions, to not make assumptions about people's histories. Generally speaking, the response to my concerns was met with disinterest; most of the time, the group did not seem that concerned. The woman who had invited me had read my report, had been at the focus-group meeting, and felt I could make a contribution.

After the first few meetings, I commented that their discussions were interesting and useful to me. They illuminated the everyday struggles of living on welfare, and I said I was excited by their resistance and analysis. This, I argued, was a form of "life skills" training, which was a common component of many required welfare programs, but in their case, they, rather than the state, were determining what issues were the focus of their problem-solving and communication efforts. I expressed my interest in documenting their discussions and activities as part of my own research into life skills training for women. Indeed, this was the theme I had hoped to explore using research funds that I had received as part of a larger network exploring the outcomes of training. Although my first plan was to study a formal training program, it struck me that working with this group was another way to continue my research into women's learning processes. I showed them a summary of my proposal and the ethical consent forms, and the group agreed to participate. "You use us and we use you" was the response by the group leader. I also discussed this shift in the site of my research with the main principal investigator of the network, who agreed that this was a great opportunity.

I then asked the women what kind of resources I could contribute, and so, using my research budget, I began to pay for lunches and coffees when we met at a local coffee shop. I also gave them funds for child care, so they could attend meetings. The issue of nutrition was often a concern, and when

I asked what I could do (besides making the government raise the IA rates), they asked me to bring food that they could take home to their families. So began my ritual of Costco® shopping trips to buy frozen meat products like sausages, chicken fingers, meat, and pies (they had asked for these items) which I brought to the meetings and distributed. At another time, they talked about not being able to afford to buy dictionaries for their personal use and to help with their children's homework. This was considered a luxury and beyond their budget. I bought them all hard-cover English dictionaries, and the women were thrilled to each take one home. I had some limited funds for computer and Internet training, and two of the group members indicated an interest; I bought them new computers and found a colleague to give them some basic assistance with Internet training. I also brought research articles on topics that the group was discussing. Sometimes the women called these meetings "Women's Studies 101." I submitted my receipts for remuneration, naming them as workshop and outreach expenses; there were no questions asked about these expenses.

I continued to be self-conscious of my different class location, while it seemed at times that the others were less concerned. Social class differences, however, did arise. During one meeting, we were having a discussion about safety, and I commented on how safety means different things to different people. One member of the group was nodding her head vigorously, and then she spoke about how she felt safe when she had left her husband who used to repeatedly beat her. The direct way she spoke of her many years of violence was shocking to me. I felt guilty that my life had been so easy, and I was embarrassed sharing what felt like a banal experience. From these meetings, I learned an enormous amount about the lived reality of poverty and how it affected all aspects of these women's lives. I also reflected on how many of their encounters were with problems that I had never had to deal with. For example, the women were concerned about their children's health, but felt that they were under surveillance every time they took their children to a doctor or medical clinic. They worried about these visits being used by the state as an excuse to take the children away; they had heard stories of this happening. They spoke about problems with landlords who wouldn't deal with repairs, who would charge them $50 to replace a lost key. They couldn't afford this, so when they lost their keys, they simply left their places unlocked, all the time worrying about break-ins. Many spoke about how they would love to move to better living quarters; the social housing they were in was cheaply put together and cramped, and some of their children had allergies which they felt were related to their housing situations. If they did find a better place, they likely wouldn't get their down payments back, or be able to afford a new one, or have their moving costs covered by welfare.

They talked about having to go long distances on the bus with their children to fill in forms for services for which they were eligible. Those taking courses to complete their high school or a post-secondary credential talked about how hard it was to concentrate and study, worrying about their child care arrangements (or trying to study when their children needed attention) and falling behind in their studies when their kids were sick. When they were telling most of these stories, I was struck by how punitive welfare reform and below-poverty benefits had created these struggles. I wanted to make a difference but often felt very limited in my capacity to bring about change. Some of my knowledge, however, was useful. Working in the post-secondary system, I offered advice on how to negotiate the bureaucracy for one participant, who was going to quit a course and thus receive a failing grade on her transcript. She felt she couldn't write the mid-term exam because she had fallen behind because of child care demands. I suggested that she write the exam, even without studying, and commented that she might know more than she realized; she did write the exam and passed the course with strong marks. She referred to this moment as a significant shift in her regard for her intellectual abilities and a moment when she began to think of alternative pathways. After I had begun to bring frozen meat to the meetings, one woman noticed that she found she could study much better after she started getting more protein. This was another moment when I was struck by the social class differences between myself and this group; I had never experienced problems because of malnutrition.

Working across the Class Divide

I heard many stories about dealing with the middle-class biases of store-keepers, bus drivers, welfare workers, health care workers, academic researchers, and schools. I realized the gap between my everyday world and theirs, and my sense that we lived in different cultures was deepened. They spoke about attending local community meetings and finding that they were often the only people receiving welfare or who routinely struggled to make ends meet. At one meeting, it had been suggested that a useful strategy to help the poor would be to collect recipes for soup that would only cost a few pennies to make. The women spoke up at these kinds of meetings, expressing their frustration with the ideas being raised. Did they not think lone mothers on welfare didn't know every trick in the book to make inexpensive meals? Did they not see that if they really wanted to help, they should join others in a movement to raise welfare rates? The group members talked about how expressing anger made people upset and uncomfortable, how they were to suppress their frustrations and be grateful.

The women in the group were very knowledgeable about the rules and regulations and took it upon themselves to help others. The group leader, who had wanted a computer and Internet training, was becoming so proficient at Web-based searches and finding information that she was helping others in her housing complex fill in forms, find out their rights, and contact the proper agencies. Group members went with their neighbours to the welfare office and helped them get emergency food vouchers or other resources to which they were entitled. They talked about how to be effective in these encounters, coming in fully informed of the rules and what they could ask for, taking notes, and asking for names of workers, while staying calm and polite, but assertive.

At one point, I raised the prospect of conducting interviews with other women in the housing complex, suggesting that this research could be useful for their advocacy efforts. There was some cautious interest, so I brought some initial questions for discussion. The questions were thoroughly critiqued. I remember feeling embarrassed (again) when they pointed out the middle-class bias of the questions and how they missed capturing much of the daily struggle of living in poverty. In the end, we rejected the idea of these interviews; it would mean asking questions and prying into women's lives. When receiving welfare benefits, women already had enough of that experience. Why would women want to sit and talk about their struggles, about how depressing it was to not have enough money to feed their children?

At various times in the meetings, I would ask the group if they were still comfortable with my participation. I shared drafts of writing I had done about the lives of lone mothers on welfare. Some of these papers reflected the group's discussions, and they gave useful feedback. Several members of the group joined me at a policy workshop on welfare reform, where we presented a statement of principles; they were the only people in the room who had any experience with the system. I co-authored a paper with the group leader, and we co-presented at a conference that was funded by a community-university research network. I wanted to show her the environment in which I worked and to have her recognized as a co-author (Boggan and Butterwick 2004). While many of the conference papers were about welfare, as with my earlier experience, my co-presenter, Amanda Boggan, was the only person present who was receiving income assistance. At these meetings, the academic audience was very polite. The question directing the conference papers was "What outcomes matter to you?" and when she answered that question from her lived reality, her response did not fit with expectations. We both noticed a subtle shift when some other academics were asking her questions, whereby she became an object of their inquiry, not a subject of her own life or a co-investigator of our research. We debriefed after that event, and she shared her observations about the middle-class orientation and abstract discourse. It made me reflect on how there were moments when I, too, had shifted in my relationship with the women in our group, moments when they became objects. They were acutely aware of these shifts and called me on them. While I was embarrassed and uncomfortable, I valued these exchanges. It seemed to me that there was enough trust and respect that they felt they could be direct and critical without the danger of me becoming defensive or leaving their project.

Generating Funds ...
After about two years, the meeting discussions shifted to raising funds to support their advocacy work. Someone suggested making gift baskets that the group would put together and sell. This was met with great enthusiasm, and so gift baskets were created consisting of homemade preserves, chocolates, and scones; recipes for the homemade items; plus a mug filled with coffee and tea packages. Each basket had a small card inserted that explained the group and its goals. The name of the group generated a heated discussion: they decided to name themselves the Poor Women's Collective; however, this title was not welcomed by all members. Various recipes were tested and comparative shopping ventures were undertaken. Putting their limited funds together, these women were able to purchase some wholesale products. We learned about pricing and marketing, turning recipes for small batches of jam and scones into ones for bulk cooking, about working cooperatively, and about using the computer to make labels and to print information about the group.

When this initiative started, I began to feel more useful. I helped by looking for and buying some of these items and putting the baskets together. I also took on the role of seller, as I had access to people with money, although some of the women sold a few baskets themselves. I brought them to work, conferences, and various meetings and sold them to my academic colleagues and friends. Making these baskets and selling them made me feel much more of an equal participant.

The baskets were beautiful creations, carefully pulled together with hours of labour. Some group members commented on the contrast between these carefully crafted high-quality baskets and their everyday lived experiences of searching for the cheapest food and living frugally, without frills – such as special teas, coffees, and homemade jams! While the group was quite energized during these activities, there was also conflict and some tensions, as some felt they were doing more work than others. Cracks began to appear in the group. As hopes were raised by the basket sales, the group began to wonder if this might be a way to generate income, not just for their organization, but as a business that could help them become economically independent. And so more gift baskets were made and taken to flea markets; tables were purchased at craft fairs, where these baskets were put on sale. Few sales were made at these venues, but I continued to sell them to my friends and colleagues, who seemed quite happy to support the group in this way. Given the welfare regulations of declaring all income, which would then be taken off their welfare payments, I was given all of the sales money, and I opened a new account under my name. At one point, there was over $1,000, which was a large amount of savings for this group.

The women in the group began to expand their ideas about what could go into the gift baskets. In this next venture, they explored the world of import and export, fair trade, and communication with women's co-operatives in Central America. The group leader, now a savvy Internet surfer, had made connections with some non-profit organizations in the United States and Central America. From these links, she identified several co-operatives in Central America, where the women were involved in handmade crafts. Samples of these items were purchased, but many did not survive the journey through the regular postal service. Courier services were used for the next shipment, which arrived safely. New materials, including ceramic bowls and cups, wooden carvings, handmade shorts, and earrings made their way to the group, and new gift baskets were created using these products.

This time the women priced the baskets significantly higher, reflecting the costs of purchasing, shipping, and their own labour. While my colleagues had readily purchased the earlier "tea break baskets," indicating that they thought they were attractive and that they wanted to support the project, they found the higher-priced baskets too expensive. We made few sales of these new baskets. The women in the group had many discussions about marketing and pricing, and they realized that they could not compete with other non-profit organizations such as Oxfam that had set up stores and catalogue businesses to sell similar items.

Other collective income-generating options were also explored, including running a day care centre and thrift store. I rented a van and took most of the women and their children to Victoria, where we visited such an establishment, meeting with the co-operative and hearing about their challenges and successes. While there was a great need for the centre, they struggled to get government funding and, in the end, could not generate enough money to leave welfare. Continuing with the idea of reselling used things, I went to a warehouse outside of Victoria with the group leader to explore the important-export business of used blue jeans. The only way to make any money, we were told, was to undertake a massive project, which was outside of the group's capacity.

The next project they explored was creating a Web-based catalogue, where other non-profit groups could purchase space to sell their handmade crafts. Research was conducted over a period of months, including explorations of various Web design software, acquiring the capacity to accept credit cards over the Internet, and exploring security issues related to credit payments on the Internet. At this point, the women became very interested in the notion of fair trade and discovered, using the Internet, a variety of organizations involved with developing fair trade principles and evaluating companies for fair trade certification. Connections were made with a local Latin American advocacy group, and a new territory of importing goods was explored, that of bringing in fair trade organic coffee. To avoid the problems with the postal service experienced earlier on and the high costs of a courier, the group partnered with someone who drove down to Central America and returned with the coffee as well as other crafts made by several women's co-operatives. On the way through the United States, the truck was stopped and seized by immigration authorities, and the driver was put in jail. Members of the group became involved in organizing, mainly on the Internet, to have the driver and truck released. Eventually, the driver was freed, but the truck and its contents never were returned, and so the group lost their products and their investment.

A Developing Friendship
After a couple of years of selling baskets and exploring the idea of a Web-based fair trade co-operative and other possibilities, the group had begun to lose members, and it finally dissolved. Some of the women had found jobs;

others had moved to different areas to live. The funds I'd been keeping were divided up among the members. I continued to meet with the group leader, who had now began in earnest to finish her undergraduate degree through distance courses, and we became friends. She had a learning disability that created problems; I found a colleague at the university who undertook an assessment, which was forwarded to the welfare system. We hoped she would be able to get disability benefits, and thus not have to start looking for work, as her youngest child was soon turning three and under the regulations at the time she would have to do so. The assessment, while conducted by a recognized professional psychologist, was unfortunately not accepted. I learned a great deal about the politics of applying for disability benefits from her struggles for recognition.

At that time, recipients of income assistance could get an extra $100 a month if they volunteered for forty hours a week. This seemed highly exploitative, given that people on welfare would likely seize this opportunity to bring in some extra income. Furthermore, the hourly wage was $4, certainly a signal to recipients of how their labour was of little value. That said, the group leader discussed this policy, and in the end I "hired" her as a community researcher, which required that I fill in monthly forms as her "employer" and send them to her welfare worker so that she could get these extra funds. The research she conducted was to document her experiences of distance learning (she was working on completing her degree through the Open Learning Agency). I also managed to have her take a directed studies course with me on that topic, which involved quite a significant amount of bureaucratic manoeuvring (undergraduate students usually cannot take graduate courses). As a faculty member, I was also able to get her a library card as a community researcher, under my name. For that directed study course, she explored the academic discussions on distance education and self-directed learning and wrote her final paper pointing to the middle-class assumptions inherent in the literature, which opened my eyes even further to the biases of other elements in my field.

We met monthly, I often took her and her two preschool children out to lunch, and we wrote almost daily via e-mail. She completed her degree, and we celebrated with a dinner at my house. I continued connecting with her as she applied (with a reference from me) to an online master's program in creative non-fiction. She had been writing stories about her experiences and thought she might be able to publish them. She did well in her studies but also spoke about feeling quite different from her peers, none of whom were on income assistance or knew of anyone receiving welfare.

She dropped out of the program when she became pregnant. We discussed the matter of bringing children into a world of poverty; she was adamant that she had a right to have this child and that being middle class and someone with economic resources should not be the required standard. Shortly after she had her child, the father left her, taking with him what remained of her student loan funds. I was outraged, as was she, and supported her efforts to track him down. I also struggled to understand her decision to trust this man, and this created a distance between us. Busy with her new baby, we stopped having e-mail contact, and we lost touch. I have thought of her many times since. In retrospect, I see that I made a choice to not re-engage, sensing a need to maintain some boundaries. I have felt some guilt over that decision. Much to my delight, over four years later, she recently sent me a note, commenting on how great our collaboration had been and seeking some advice about a new advocacy issue she was now working on. She also reported that she had been diagnosed with a disability that was (finally) recognized by the state, thus she was able to receive disability welfare benefits, which mean that she is not required to find work; her benefits are also higher than those in the expected-to-work category. I hope to see her again.

Reflections

In this final section, I reflect on the dialogic approach that was a key element of this project and how ongoing conversations with the group of women and the emerging relationships were shaped by social class as well as other dimensions. I consider the consciousness raising and transformative social action outcomes of this project and close with some thoughts on the paradoxical aspects of class in relation to building solidarity and achieving reciprocity.

The dialogic orientation present from the beginning was critical to achieving reciprocity. As an adult educator, I was familiar with a dialogic approach to teaching, wherein the teacher is learner and learners are also teachers, and I brought that perspective into our conversations. Being in dialogue with these women enabled a co-creative process of naming the world, a central element for Freire (1970, 89) of liberatory pedagogy, which stands in contrast to a process in which one world view dominates. This dialogue had already begun when I met with some of the women in the focus group I set up to explore themes in my summary of evaluation studies. I did not seek out this group in order to study their learning processes, rather, the opportunity to conduct research with them emerged from my community development orientation. Furthermore, time was needed to build trusting and respectful relationships; without spending considerable time with this group of women, no project would have emerged. Spending the time I did with them might be a luxury that many cannot afford, given the demands of academic work. That said, the temporal dimension of successful community-university partnerships is significant.

Dialogue, Freire argues, "must not serve as a crafty instrument for the domination of one person by another" (1970, 89). Like Freire, Lather points to the need for "praxis-oriented inquiry [in which the] reciprocal educative process is more important than product as empowering methods contribute to consciousness raising and transformative social action" (1991, 72). It is important to emphasize that while I shared many of the interests of the members of the group, their praxis was focused on finding a way to improve their lives, which involved both challenging the system and creating new opportunities for their economic survival. My praxis was oriented to my role as a feminist researcher. Furthermore, they were not particularly interested in becoming researchers, which has been identified as a "good" outcome of community-university partnerships. The women were comfortable with my agenda, but they were not going to change directions.

A dialogic orientation to feminist community-based research requires that feminist researchers critically engage with a multidimensional approach, as outlined by Naples (2003, 197): "Researchers' social positions (not limited to one's gender, race, ethnicity, class, culture, and place or region of residence)" has a bearing on the whole process. What is also significant to a dialogic orientation is an engagement with both the affective and intellectual dimensions of our being. The emotional dimensions of this project were intertwined with the intellectual. As Jo Littler points out, we need to be critically aware of "the nature of the alliances through which the individual is constituted and situated" (2005, 246). In this reflective account, the kinds of alliances that were developed were between an academic researcher and community participants. I also brought other "selves" to my encounters with these women, some present at the beginning and others which were emergent (Reinharz 1997); I was also a learner, an educator, a feminist, a friend, a confidante, as well as a purchaser and a seller.

In this project, there were elements of consciousness raising and transformative social action. In most day-to-day interactions, given where I work and live, my middle-class life does not come under scrutiny. Working collaboratively with these women, the privileges afforded to me were in stark contrast to their concerns with food, housing, and transportation, among other things. I developed a deeper understanding of the minutiae of how class inequality is structurally maintained by welfare policy and regulations, as well as by the dominant middle-class orientation that permeates everyday interactions. As Andrew Sayer notes, "one of the most important features of class inequalities is that they present people with unequal bases for respect" (2007, 99). I learned a great deal about the welfare state from the standpoint of these women's everyday experiences, a key source of knowledge, and one emphasized by Dorothy Smith (1987). Taking up the standpoint of women, in Smith's view, means an examination of "relations, practices, powers, and forces which are actual," most particularly, social class, given its centrality to a process of "explicating the actual organization of relations in which our lives and struggles are embedded" (44).

The women in the group also learned, particularly when I brought some feminist literature to our discussions of the welfare state. Reading this literature echoed their own analysis and thus confirmed their abilities for critical thinking; the women also expressed surprise at the level of attention by academic researchers given to them. Developing a deeper understanding of the structural dimensions of their everyday struggles was, for some, a significant shift. The group leader also learned, through our partnership, about the limits and points of access to post-secondary education. In relation to creating social change, this project taught me a great deal about limitations as well as possibilities and the importance of working the space between. This project challenged the class divide and built a bridge between the university and this particular community. Furthermore, documenting and participating in this group's activism contributed in some way to supporting what Fraser calls "subaltern counter publics," which are "parallel discursive arenas where members of subordinated social groups invent and circulate counter discourses" (1997, 81).

In some sense, this collaborative project speaks to how feminist community-based research can subvert repressive state processes, most particularly, those processes that expect silence, compliance, and gratitude from individuals receiving welfare. In contrast, this project valued these women's activism, their voice, their analysis, and their resistance to these mechanisms. As bell hooks notes, we need "more written work and oral testimony documenting ways barriers are broken down, coalitions formed and solidarity shared" (1994, 110).

My growing collegial friendship, particularly with the group leader, was an unexpected development. I was delighted that she was interested in co-authoring some papers, and I felt that my support of her hopes to further

her education was a significant form of reciprocity. Stacey, however, points to the dangers of these alliances, arguing that "fieldwork represents an intrusion and intervention into a system of relationships, a system of relationship that the researcher is far freer than the researched to leave" (1991, 113). Given the dialogic orientation and time devoted to this project, I would not characterize my engagement as an intrusion or an intervention. After the group leader's third child was born, our communication lapsed for some years; we reconnected after several years had passed. It seems that there was some mutuality in the initial decision to let the friendship go. It should be noted, however, that, at least from my perspective, I entered her life much more than she entered mine, a situation that had much to do with our social class differences. I had also become, to a certain extent, part of her social network, and it is possible that my disengagement created problems for her. The ethics of purposefully developing this kind of intimacy within our research projects does need to be considered. Now that I have renewed communication with the group leader, I have an opportunity to explore these concerns and the notion of reciprocity further.

I will conclude my reflections by noting some of the challenges and paradoxes of reciprocity. Iris Marion Young suggests that we can only achieve "asymmetrical reciprocity"; we can move beyond our immediate standpoints but we can never know "the standpoint of the other person ... only into a mediated relationship between us" (1997, 47). Razack offers further insight into the challenges of achieving reciprocity, particularly when working across class differences: "To reach each other across our differences or to resist patriarchal and racist constructs, we must overcome at least one difficulty: the difference in position between the teller and the listener, between telling the tale and hearing it" (1998, 36). While I argue that significant levels of reciprocity were achieved in this project, class and other "dis-stances" (Fine 1994) were always mediating our relationships.

Another challenge of this project was balancing the time spent "in the field" with producing publications, a requirement for maintaining an academic position. A dialogic approach, as noted by Freire and Lather, emphasizes process over product, which created challenges for me during my tenure and promotion process, something I have written about elsewhere (Butterwick and Dawson 2005). Creating those products that are valued by the academy is a requirement to staying in the academy, and staying in the academy brings access to many resources, both material and discursive. In other words, I doubt I would have embarked on this journey if I did not have an academic position. I would advise others interested in similar kinds of projects to recognize this paradox and work more effectively within this tension and the duality of their work. Effective feminist community-based research requires that we be aware of our stance and our "dis-stance." As Fine notes, "all researchers are agents in the flesh (Caraway, 1991) and in the collective, who choose, wittingly or not, from among a controversial and constraining set of political stances and epistemologies" (1994, 16). I would further advise that feminist community-oriented researchers work with a stance of "moral humility" and "wonder," as argued by Young: "A respectful stance of wonder toward other people is one of openness across [difference], awaiting new insight about their needs, interests, perceptions or values. Wonder also means being able to see one's own position, assumptions, perspective as strange, because it has been put in relation to others" (1997, 56).

ACKNOWLEDGMENTS
I greatly appreciate the critical feedback on earlier drafts of this chapter from Gillian Creese and Paul Kershaw. The collaborative spirit of other authors has been immensely rewarding, as have been their commentaries on my chapter during our workshops.

REFERENCES
Alcoff, Linda. 1991. "The Problem of Speaking for Others." *Cultural Critique* 20: 5-32.

Boggan, A., and S. Butterwick. (2004). "Poverty, Policy and Research: Towards a Dialogic Investigation." In E. Meiners and F. Ibanez, eds., *Public Acts: Disrupting Readings on Curriculum and Research*, 113-34. New York: Routledge/Falmer.

Butterwick, S., A. Bonson, and P. Rogers. 1998. *Identifying Keys to Successful Transition from Social Assistance to Paid Work: Lessons Learned from Canada, United States, Australia and Europe*. Commissioned by Human Resources Development Canada, Vancouver, BC.

Butterwick, S., and J. Dawson. 2005. "Simplest Things Last: Examining the Production of Academic Labour." *Women's Studies International Forum* 28: 51-65.

Carragata, L. 2003. "Neoconservative Realities: The Social and Economic Marginalization of Canadian Women." *International Sociology* 18(3): 559-80.

Fine, Michelle. 1994. "Dis-tances and Other Stances: Negotiations of Power inside Feminist Research." In A. Gitlin, ed., *Power and Method: Political Activism and Educational Research*, 13-35. New York: Routledge.

Freire, Paulo. 1970. *Pedagogy of the Oppressed*. New York: Continuum.

Fraser, Nancy. 1997. *Justice Interruptus: Critical Reflections on the Postsocialist Condition*. New York: Routledge.

hooks, bell. 1994. *Teaching to Transgress: Education as the Practice of Freedom*. New York: Routledge.

Lather, Patti. 1991. *Getting Smart: Feminist Research and Pedagogy with/in the Postmodern.* New York: Routledge.

Littler, Jo. 2005. "Beyond the Boycott Anti-Consumerism, Cultural Change and the Limits of Reflexivity." *Cultural Studies* 19(2): 227-52.

Naples, N. 2003. *Feminism and Method: Ethnography, Discourse Analysis, and Activist Research.* New York: Routledge.

Nesbit, T. 2005. "Social Class and Adult Education." In T. Nesbit, ed., *Class Concerns: Adult Education and Social Class,* 5-14. New Directions for Adult and Continuing Education, Issue 106. New York: Wiley.

Razack, Sherene. 1998. *Looking White People in the Eye: Gender, Race and Culture in Courtrooms and Classrooms.* Toronto: University of Toronto Press.

Reinharz, Shulamit. (1997) "Who Am I? The Need for a Variety of Selves in the Field." In R. Hertz, ed., *Reflexivity and Voice,* 3-20. Thousand Oaks, CA: Sage.

Sayer, Andrew. 2007. "Class, Moral Worth and Recognition." In T. Lovell, ed., *(Mis)recognition, Social Inequality and Social Justice: Nancy Fraser and Pierre Bourdieu,* 88-102. New York: Routledge.

Smith, Dorothy. 1987. *The Everyday World as Problematic: A Feminist Sociology.* Toronto: University of Toronto Press.

Stacey, Judith. 1991. "Can There Be a Feminist Ethnography?" In S.B. Gluck and B. Patai, eds., *Women's Words: The Feminist Practice of Oral History,* 111-20. New York: Routledge.

Young, Iris Marion. 1990. *Justice and the Politics of Difference.* Princeton, NJ: Princeton University Press.

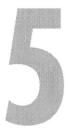

Voices from the Street
Sex Workers' Experiences in
Community-Based HIV Research

JILL CHETTIAR, MARK W. TYNDALL,
KATHARINE CHAN, DEVI PARSAD,
KATE GIBSON, AND KATE SHANNON

Background

Increasing numbers of women exchange sex for money, drugs, or other goods for the purpose of day-to-day survival on the streets across Canada. Globally, survival sex workers continue to experience higher rates of violence, poverty, drug-related harms, physical and mental ill health, stigma, and discrimination that likely elevate their risk of HIV infection and other sexually transmitted infections (STIs) and mortality (El-Bassel et al. 2001; Romero-Daza, Weeks, and Singer 2003; Shannon et al. 2005, 2007; Shannon, Kerr, Bright et al. 2008). In Canada, initial research in major urban centres suggests that women who exchange sex for survival and use drugs are increasingly vulnerable to HIV infection. The World Health Organization currently estimates that less than 15 percent of sex workers worldwide have adequate access to prevention resources. Given that lack of access to prevention remains the strongest predictor of HIV transmission, understanding the individual, social, and structural contexts of vulnerability among sex workers remains critical in ensuring improved prevention, treatment, and support for this population.

Sex Work Environment in Canada

While the exchange of money for sex has always been legal in Canada, sex work exists in a largely prohibitive environment. In particular, the communicating provision (negotiation between sex workers and clients in public

spaces), the procuring and the bawdy-house provisions (operating a common bawdy house, private spaces) in Canada's Criminal Code make it
largely impossible for sex workers to operate legally (PIVOT, Sex-Work
Committee 2004). Evidence has increasingly shown that the consequences
of these laws and enforcement-based practices are to further criminalize the
sex industry and force the most vulnerable sex workers engaged in survival
sex to work in isolated and unsanitary public spaces away from health,
prevention, and support services (Lowman 2000; Goodyear et al. 2005;
Shannon, Kerr, Allinott et al. 2008; Shannon, Strathdee, Shoveller et al.
2009). Over the last decade, the street-level sex industry in Vancouver,
British Columbia, has received significant media coverage, with the high-
profile missing and murdered women and subsequent arrest and trial of the
largest serial murderer in Canadian history.[1] Unfortunately, despite over
$116 million spent on the trial and extensive focus on the social contexts and
harms experienced by women in survival sex work in Vancouver, alarming
rates of adverse health outcomes such as STIs, including HIV (Spittal et al.
2002; Weber et al. 2002; Shannon et al. 2005; Shannon, Kerr, Bright et al.
2008) persist. Increased risk of sexual assault was found to be linked to
such structural factors as homelessness and criminalization of the sex work
environment – specifically, policing strategies that push sex workers away
from main streets (Shannon, Kerr, Strathdee et al. 2009).

WISH and the Development of the Maka Project
In response, in late 2004 service providers and board members of the
Women's Information Safe Haven (WISH) Drop-In Centre Society and researchers at the BC Centre for Excellence in HIV/AIDS partnered to undertake an initial needs assessment of health-related harms and barriers to
prevention and care for women in survival sex work (Shannon et al. 2005).
WISH is a drop-in centre that had been operating in Vancouver's inner city
community, the Downtown Eastside, since 1987, providing a safe space and
meals for sex workers. WISH has since become a hub of activity, running a
variety of support, health, safety, and pre-employment programs for sex
workers. The results of initial surveys conducted in 2003 were concerning:
just over a quarter of women surveyed tested positive for HIV, and only
9 percent of HIV-positive women were on highly active anti-retroviral treatment (HAART). A further cause for concern was the knowledge that the
study was limited to women who were already at least accessing services at
WISH – there were likely women in the community at even higher risk of

infection whom researchers and service providers had no apparent ways to access. The results of this initial work led to the inception of a formal community-based HIV research partnership, the Maka Project.

As described in detail elsewhere (Shannon et al. 2007), a key component of the project was capacity building among a team of women in survival sex work, supported by an open Community Advisory Board (CAB) that informed all stages of the project. The hiring process developed by the CAB aimed to ensure that the entire process was transparent and easily accessible to women in a variety of life situations. Project staff, in concert with the CAB, made efforts to offer extensive and flexible options for women to contact the project (outreach, community agency visits, open house for women) and the creation of a community-peer hiring panel (CAB members). Through this process, a team of women with a lived experience of survival sex work were hired, trained, and supported to play an active role in guiding, developing, and conducting the research. Low-threshold employment positions were designed from a harm reduction perspective, based on lessons learned and shared by community-sex-worker and drug-user groups. There was considerable focus on capacity building and training, as well as ongoing support and referral for addictions counselling, drug treatment, supportive housing, and child care. Training was developed and delivered in collaboration with community agencies and service providers, including local sex work organizations such as Prostitution Alternatives, Counselling, and Education (PACE) Society. Sessions on lateral oppression, vicarious trauma, debriefing, and conflict resolution; participatory action research principles, methodologies, ethics, and informed consent; and health, HIV/HCV prevention, and harm reduction were offered and, when possible, conducted or co-facilitated by sex worker groups, community services providers, or Aboriginal agencies (Shannon et al. 2007).

Using social mapping, peer-administered interview questionnaires, and focus groups co-facilitated by sex workers and academic researchers, the objective of the study was to see where gaps existed in HIV prevention and harm reduction services for women, and to find out from the women themselves how best to fill these gaps. Peer workers were tasked with conducting one-on-one questionnaire-based interviews and social-mapping sessions. Outreach and recruitment activities had teams of peer and non-experiential researchers seeking new participants at different times of day and night throughout the City of Vancouver. Additionally, peer workers who were interested in doing so received further training and co-facilitated focus groups with specific research themes (e.g., policing, use of condoms, access to HIV treatment). While the conception, design, and methodology of this community-based research project have been discussed in further detail elsewhere (Shannon et al. 2007), this qualitative process and impact evaluation examines the narratives and reflective experiences of survival sex workers as peer researchers in the project.

Reflecting on Community-Based Research

In this chapter, we undertake to examine the impacts of participatory-action research methods on community members involved in the implementation of the study. Further, we wish to problematize the concept of "peerness" and the use of the word *peer* as a signifier of both similarity and difference in the context of this community-based research project. Examining these themes in a focus group discussion, we wish to explore the meaning of participation in participatory action research for non-academic researchers.

As this is a community-based research project, it is important to define our community. Certainly, the idea of community and how it is defined has no clear or singular answer: rather than choose to define the study's target population by geographical location, recent experience in Vancouver's sex trade was the defining parameter with a focus on street-based solicitation. Our project office was located in the Downtown Eastside (DTES), an area of the city that has high concentrations of drug use and survival sex work, as well as low-threshold health and social services. A significant portion of our constructed community would turn out to be tied in some way to the DTES, but we made efforts to extend the boundaries of the research site. By recruiting at various times of the day and night on active strolls all over the city and through the use of alternative study locations (e.g., hotel rooms, community centres), we were able to extend beyond the immediate surroundings of the project office. Time-location sampling, mapping of solicitation spaces, and targeted outreach with the assistance of service providers increased access to hard-to-reach members of the study's researched community.

Methods

The Maka Project was conceptualized, developed, implemented, and disseminated through a process of co-construction of knowledge in the negotiated space of sex workers and community and academic partners (Shannon et al. 2007). This negotiated space, the "sociosanitary space," seeks to confront and reduce power imbalances, and it is a process inherent in participatory action research and public health partnerships with marginalized populations (Bernier et al. 2006). The research was both guided and theoretically influenced by feminist-driven PAR. In particular, the research process aimed to challenge conventional understanding of power and power relations through empowerment, knowledge co-construction, and the validation of "lived experiences" of sex workers as knowledge (Reason 1994; Shannon, Kerr, Allinott et al. 2008). It has been suggested that this transdisciplinary dialogue can propose new ends to public health, rather than applying standardized solutions to health disparities by outside experts (Bernier et al. 2006).

Importantly, while PAR is increasingly adopted as an approach to HIV research, there remain critical gaps in examining how PAR is experienced and interpreted by the community involved in the project. In an effort to examine the process and the impact of the Maka Project as a community-based HIV research project on women working as peer researchers, we conducted a focus group discussion with the peer research team. Women who were currently employed as peer workers with the Maka Project were invited to participate in a focus group discussion, facilitated by the first author (JC). Everyone was informed of the topic in advance – their experience as peer workers in general, and as peer workers at Maka specifically. Six women were invited, and five attended. The women who participated ranged in age from twenty-three to forty-five years, and of the women who attended, three were Aboriginal. Collectively, the women have decades of experience in various aspects of the sex trade (primarily street-based sex work) in mainly urban settings throughout western Canada. Food and drink were supplied, as well as an honorarium of $25 for their expertise and time. This research received ethical approval under the University of British Columbia/Providence Health Research Ethics Review Board, and was also reviewed by the PACE Society sex work research and policy committee.

As the discussion began, the women were a bit reticent. This was an unusual situation, as the women involved in the focus group were habituated to being in the interviewer role within the confines of the Maka Project. The sudden role reversal – interviewers becoming interviewees within the same project – was initially a bit strained. However, once the conversation was underway, the women were more at ease and opened up to share their opinions and reflections on their experiences and their roles in the Maka Project.

Results

Community-Based Research Methods as Interventions

A key theme that emerged during the focus group discussion was the impact on the women of the experience as peer workers. During the process of constructing the research design and foci, the emphasis was completely on the process itself and how it could directly benefit both individual participants and the community at large. In the focus group discussion with the Maka workers, it became apparent that there was another layer of potential benefits – to the peer workers themselves. Throughout the focus group discussion, the women referred to ways in which working at the Maka Project had changed how they saw themselves:

> It [being a peer worker] has given me more confidence.

> I think I'm more of a role model. Some people give me positive compliments. In the beginning, at the end of the survey, it felt weird to have people thank me.

In addition, the women described more than once instances where their work with the Maka Project had provided either the financial support, structure, or peer support needed to make some changes in their routines, particularly pertaining to drug use and/or sex work:

> It [being a peer worker] has given me more of an incentive to get my shit together. Now I have a home over my head, I have a phone, I can pay for my bills, I have cable, I'm not working 24/7, shooting up 24/7. It has shown me the direction I've always wanted to go towards but couldn't. Gave me that initiative to get the ball rolling. Anything is attainable if you believe in it.

> Before I would go out seven days a week, even in the afternoons unless I'm sleeping. Now I go out once a week. I just don't feel I need to do that anymore. I just feel I'm at a different place and time in my life. The drug scene's come to an end. It's time to move on; I don't want to live here forever. I'm just more comfortable to know that drugs aren't such a big part of life anymore. I don't crave it even if I see it. Having methadone is such a godsend.

> I don't work anymore because of it [being a peer worker]. I have different ideas of how I want to spend my time, different goals, and my whole mindset's changed. I'm not using drugs anymore. Once you stop using drugs, the work just disappears.

Certainly, there was no expectation that participating as peer workers would cause harm, but the benefits, as described by the women themselves, went beyond the benefits expected (i.e., skills gained in training, financial compensation). Although this anecdotal evidence leads us to believe that there was a decrease in drug use and general street involvement, we are unable to compare the peer workers' day-to-day lives before and after the Maka Project. In designing future projects, an explicitly stated internal focus would be worthwhile, coupled with the development of methods that would allow closer examination of the effects of community-based research on those community members most actively engaged in administering the research.

Peer Research

One of the major ways in which community-based research seeks to be accessible to participants is by incorporating members of the target population into the research team. As previously mentioned, the Maka Project has women who do sex work involved at nearly every level, most prominently at the level of conducting and shaping the research. The term *peer* is often used in research and community organizing when members of the community are engaged and involved in the implementation of the planned activities. Using this term typically indicates that those denoted as peers are closer in experience to the target population than the academic researchers. In the research context, where the traditional extractive model of academic research is still the norm, *peer* is a stronger signifier of *less difference* than of *greater similarity*.

However, there is an implicit assumption of a community's homogeneity in the use of the word *peer* – a term that intimates a level of equality or sameness. Assumptions of homogeneity, especially when attempting to address the needs of marginalized communities, can be dangerous. In the attempt to flatten complex communities into one or more discrete categories, there is an extremely high risk that those who are marginal to these simpler, constructed categories may be rendered silent or invisible. This being said, in the context of the Maka Project (or any other project or program), there is a utility to the terminology. In fact, the necessity for such a label is most accurately framed as a problem of demarcation: there is a need to differentiate between the academic researchers and the community researchers. As *peer* is colloquially accepted and understood to express this difference in the Downtown Eastside (researchers/target population; clients/service providers), the term was employed in the Maka Project. Specifically, *peerness* was designated along lines of being experiential (in this context, having experience as street-level sex workers). While researchers recognize that this experience does not define the women involved, this was the important common ground that was necessary to establish the distinction between researchers and participants, and the key distinction to be communicated between academic and community researchers.

The common experiences between peer interviewers and study participants was viewed as necessary in making participants more comfortable in sharing their experiences with someone who had "been there and done that." In other words, this particular aspect of the design was predicated on two things: establishing a safer space for participants by lessening the power differential between researchers and researchees; and, hopefully, reducing the social desirability bias in the responses from women – the idea being that there is less pressure to lie or to "present well" when they know that the women asking the questions have had similar experiences to theirs.

It became evident through our focus group discussion that the social stratification within the community of sex workers is more complicated than the simple dichotomy of experiential/non-experiential suggests. Factors such as active drug use and condom use are sites of social scrutiny among sex workers, and divulging one's status to a perceived peer could make women feel compromised or overexposed. This highlights exactly the problem of peerness raised previously. If we can agree that identities are complex, constituted entities – so we can agree that the notion of parity even within this discrete community is never completely attainable. Recognizing this impossibility, peerness must be eschewed as a goal; rather, we must look at the social dynamics at play, recognizing that while a PAR approach addresses a specific and overarching power differential in the research context, there are other micro-level hierarchies that demand attention, albeit on a case-by-case basis. Although the level of shared experience has increased, it is possible that the relative anonymity provided by the distance between a sex worker and non-experiential interviewer can also be used by the sex worker as a protection against this exposure. Based on the discussion with the Maka peer workers, it seems that the model of peer interviewing works. Procedures at the study site were in place to avoid situations where peer workers were interviewing family, friends, or close acquaintances. However, reflecting on their past work, the peer workers clearly identified a grey area – women who they perhaps did not know personally, but who were not completely anonymous to them (since they had seen them on strolls, in the community, etc.):

I don't think it [being a peer worker] was a barrier, I think it depended on whether they knew you or not.

They're comfortable because they know we're not an authority figure.

Inclusivity

In carrying out a peer researcher–based research project, there are many challenges that must be surmounted. There is an inherent division between the researchers behind the project and the women they wish to engage as peer employees and, later, as research participants. Of course, one of the central ideas behind community-based participatory action research is recognition of this divide, and conscious attempts are made to narrow the gap. However, the gap is never completely eliminated, and we run the risk of defeating our own purposes in not carefully acknowledging the space between us, while negotiating closer relationships throughout the project.

Inclusivity is a key concept in bringing researchers and participants closer together. Clearly, creating peer researcher positions is one of the major modes of including the community being researched in the process of research itself. It is important, then, to consult these peers about the degree to which they themselves felt included – for it is easy enough to create token positions of access to the community that signify inclusion without actually following through.

Therefore, this theme was one that was probed in our focus group with the Maka Project peer workers. Throughout the focus group, examples of specific instances of inclusion were named, in addition to a general sense of belonging and openness, which (based on the feedback from the peers) seemed to have been principally communicated through the creation of a non-coercive, non-punitive working environment and training regimen:

> [regarding training] It was easy because they show you what you have to do, and if you get it wrong, nobody gives you shit. You just feel you should pay more attention to what you were doing. I didn't think it was stressful at all.

Women had the impression from the very beginning of their involvement with the Maka Project, which is to say, beginning with the hiring process, that this was a space where they would not be judged for participation in sex work or for drug use:

> [regarding interview process] The only part that surprised me was that they didn't ask me about my current situation. I guess I was expecting they

would ask me if I was still working and if I was still using. I guess I thought that if they knew I was still working I wouldn't really make a good candidate ... They weren't judgmental. It really alleviated the weight I had on my shoulders about coming there.

Reflexivity

This inclusivity created the necessary environment for reflexivity in the project. If women did not feel that they were integral and inherent parts of the research structure and design, we could not hope for a genuine effort at soliciting feedback on research direction or practice. We created several channels for receiving feedback about the research that had been done to date. As it turned out, these also managed to be opportunities for women to communicate with the project about the changing reality for women on the street.

Many peer workers continued to engage in sex work while they were employed at the Maka Project. They were able to feed this perspective directly into the work they were doing at the Maka Project at moments when we were designing new focus groups, or revisiting the quantitative questionnaire:

> It was pretty cool they asked for our opinions and they wanted our input on it.

> One thing I liked with the questionnaires was that every six months, we would sit with Kate, and we would go through the whole questionnaires and talk about what we thought wasn't so appropriate and what we thought should be included. So we would be ready for the next questionnaire that came up.

The efforts made to include women in the research process and research environment had the secondary function of reflexivity:

> A lot of the decision making with the program, it was a collaborative effort. It wasn't like "this is how you do it." They listened to what we had to say. A lot of times, it's like they listen to what you say but it goes in one ear and out the other. But they implemented our different ideas. They believed in us and our experience that we were going to be an asset, and it was a collaborative decision on a lot of things. It made a big difference to how I felt working here. I didn't feel like I had bosses, like I worked with a team of people.

By constantly being aware of the division between institutional researchers and peer researchers, we were able to successfully negotiate a space that was inclusive and at once fulfilled the research methodology. In many ways, this speaks to the very roots of feminist methodology and the need for reflexivity. Because we are constantly discovering more about the lives of hidden and marginalized populations, the research process itself is necessarily iterative.

The need for reflexivity in a project such as this stems, in part, from the division between the academic researchers (authors of this chapter) of the project and the research participants and peer researchers. The intention to include is surely noble, but it runs the risk of being hollow, as well. By making the research design itself a function of the inclusivity (through reflexive processes), we are able to increase the degree to which the project can truly be considered participatory.

The community-based research methods used by the Maka Project embody many of the principles of feminist research methodology. As previously mentioned, many of these were in mind as the protocol was written – others developed organically over time, sometimes through necessity and more often out of respect for the community of highly stigmatized and marginalized women that the project was accessing. In addition, many of the women involved at the investigator, Community Advisory Board, and peer worker levels were women who had been involved in research previously. Therefore, they provided an unexpected expertise and perspective, bringing their own experiences as research subjects with them to the other side of the table.

These experiences allowed women to view the research through a critical lens. It was exceedingly important to them that their work not be in vain, nor that it be superfluous or unethical:

> I was curious who was doing the research and what they were using it for. What are they going to do with this information I gathered?

> The DTES is researched to death. Is this a waste of time? Is this actually going to be implemented into something? I didn't want to be involved in something that was going to go in a drawer.

> I wanted to make sure we found out the findings. Like we know what we do, but where does it go? What is happening?

These natural urges to engage with and lead the research process matched well with the inductive and reflexive design of the questionnaires and research foci. In between each set of interviews, the instruments were reviewed with members of peer staff as well as with the Community Advisory Board. The peers were also actively engaged in the knowledge-translation and community-dissemination activities. The objective of these reviews was to ensure that the questionnaires were reflecting the realities of women's experiences and to incorporate any new ideas that peer workers had about how questions could be more clear or could more accurately reflect the answers they were being given by women in the interviews. In this instance, another facet of the community partnership became evident: by engaging with members of the study's target population in a meaningful way at the level of research design, we were able to access their experiences as research subjects as well.

Conclusions

In examining the women's reflections on the impact of the research on their own lives, it became evident that there are ways in which the research process itself can act as an intervention with positive impacts. For the Maka workers interviewed, this seemed to be linked to having a regular work schedule and a steady supplementary income. Additionally, the training coupled with experience gained opened new doors for women elsewhere in the community:

> It gives the people who are working the streets and become peers a chance to step out of the street and do something different. It gets you slowly into something you want to do. You're not working at your own hours. You have to be responsible to a set amount of time, and you can't just leave when you want to.

Peer involvement in research among sex workers is an imperative piece of any successful future project or program – not simply from a perspective of data reliability, but also for authentic community buy-in and participation. It seems that perhaps the methodologies that have been used in the community have had the desired effect of empowerment, and women have begun internalizing the value of their lived experiences:

> Peers are viewed as a bigger asset than they ever were.

> Our experiences have some meaning. It has a lot of worth.

ACKNOWLEDGMENTS

The authors would like to thank all the women and community partners who have contributed their expertise and time to make this research project possible. We would particularly like to thank the many peers who shared their voices, expertise, energy, and time with this project, including Shari, Adrian, Candice, Rebecca, Tammy, Debbie, Laurie, Shawn, Rose, Chanel, and Sandy.

NOTE

1 As there is not space here to enumerate the hundreds of missing and murdered sex workers from Vancouver's streets, the authors of this chapter have chosen not to explicitly name the convicted serial murderer at the centre of this trial (or other perpetrators of violence against sex workers) in the body of this chapter.

REFERENCES

Bernier J., M. Rock, M. Roy, R. Bujold, and L. Potvin. 2006. "Structuring an Inter-sector Research Partnership: A Negotiated Space." *Soz Praventiv Med* 51(6): 335-44.

El-Bassel, N., S.S. Witte, T. Wada, L. Gilbert, and J. Wallance. 2001. "Correlates of Partner Violence among Female Street-Based Sex Workers: Substance Abuse, History of Childhood Abuse, and HIV Risks." *AIDS Patient Care and STDs* 15(1): 41-51.

Goodyear, M., J. Lowman, B. Fischer, and M. Green. 2005. "Prostitutes Are People Too." *Lancet* 366: 9493.

Lowman, R.J. 2000. "Violence and the Outlaw Status of (Street) Prostitution in Canada." *Violence against Women* 6(9): 987-1011.

PIVOT, Sex-Work Committee. 2004. "Voices for Dignity: A Call to End the Harms Caused by Canada's Sex Trade Laws," 1-37. Vancouver: Author. Available on-line at http://www.pivotlegal.org/Publications/Voices/index.htm.

Reason, P. 1994. "Three Approaches to Participatory Inquiry." In L.K. Denzin and N.S. Lincoln, eds., *Handbook of Qualitative Research*, 324-38. Thousand Oaks, CA: Sage.

Romero-Daza, N., M. Weeks, and M. Singer. 2003. "'Nobody Gives a Damn If I Live or Die': Violence, Drugs, and Street-Level Prostitution in Inner-City Hartford, Connecticut." *Medical Anthropology* 22(3): 233-59.

Shannon, K., V. Bright, J. Duddy, and M.W. Tyndall. 2005. "Access and Utilization of HIV Treatment and Services among Women Sex Workers in Vancouver's Downtown Eastside." *Journal of Urban Health* 82(3): 488-97.

Shannon, K., V. Bright, K. Gibson, and M.W. Tyndall. 2007. "Sexual and Drug-Related Vulnerabilities for HIV Infection among Women Engaged in Survival Sex Work in Vancouver, Canada." *Canadian Journal of Public Health* 98(6): 465-69.

Shannon, K., T. Kerr, S. Allinott, J. Chettiar, J.S. Shoveller, and M.W. Tyndall. 2008. "Social and Structural Violence and Power Relations in Mitigating HIV Risk of Drug-Using Women in Survival Sex Work." *Social Science and Medicine* 66(4): 911-21.

Shannon, K., T. Kerr, V. Bright, K. Gibson, and M.W. Tyndall. 2008. "Drug Sharing with Clients as a Risk Marker for Increased Violence and Sexual and Drug-Related Harms among Survival Sex Workers." *AIDS Care* 20(2): 228-34.

Shannon, K., T. Kerr, S.A. Strathdee, J. Shoveller, J.S. Montaner, and M.W. Tyndall. 2009. "Prevalence and Correlates of Gender-Based Violence among a Cohort of Female Sex Workers." *British Medical Journal* 339: b2939.

Shannon, K., S.A. Strathdee, J. Shoveller, M. Rusch, T. Kerr, and M.W. Tyndall. 2009. "Structural and Environmental Barriers to Condom Use Negotiation with Clients among Female Sex Workers: Implications for HIV-Prevention Strategies and Policy." *American Journal of Public Health* 99(4): 659-65.

Spittal, P.M., K.J. Craib, E. Wood, N. Laliberte, K. Li, and M.W. Tyndall. 2002. "Risk Factors for Elevated HIV Incidence Rates among Female Injection Drug Users in Vancouver." *Canadian Medical Association Journal* 166(7): 894-99.

Weber A.E., J.F. Boivin, L. Blais, N. Haley, and E. Roy. 2002. "HIV Risk Profile and Prostitution among Female Street Youths." *Journal of Urban Health* 79(4): 525-35.

Working across Race, Language, and Culture with African and Chinese Immigrant Communities

GILLIAN CREESE, XIN HUANG, WENDY FRISBY,
AND EDITH NGENE KAMBERE

This chapter draws on our experiences conducting interviews across differences of race, language, and cultures with recent immigrants in the City of Vancouver, Canada. One project explored migration experiences of sixty-one women and men in the local African community through interviews with migrants from twenty-one different countries in Africa. The other project examined the experiences of fifty Chinese immigrant women who came to Vancouver from China, Hong Kong, and Taiwan. In each case, the diverse origins of the research participants were reflected in heterogeneous language, racial, and cultural backgrounds, differences that were often paved over in processes of migration and settlement in the local context. Although we have tried to disrupt these processes of marginalization and Othering, so central to immigrant experiences in Canada, a critical eye towards our own research raises troubling questions about the difficulties of conducting feminist community research across differences and complex relations of power.

The research projects with African immigrants and Chinese women immigrants were led by principal investigators (PIs) Gillian Creese and Wendy Frisby, respectively, who are white, Canadian-born or -raised, middle-class, and unilingual English-speaking academics.[1] We were outsiders to the communities in question in many ways and occupy positions of considerable power in relation to the research participants, given our privileged social locations and control over the design and funding of the research. As feminist researchers, we were acutely aware of the methodological and ethical problems that often lead to voyeuristic accounts of the objects of research. Indeed, as principal investigators, we both felt some trepidation in undertaking these research projects precisely because of our multiple outsider statuses, even though, like France Windance Twine (2000), we eschew the problematic notion that researchers should only study people like themselves.

Both research teams included members who could, to varying degrees, be considered insiders to these communities. In all cases, the research assistants (RAs) conducting the interviews with women were female immigrants to Canada, who sometimes came from the same countries as the interviewees. Xin Huang, a PhD student from Mainland China, worked as a research assistant and project manager with Wendy. She, along with two other research assistants, Hui-Ling Lin, a PhD student from Taiwan, and Sheena Yang, a PhD student from Mainland China, conducted interviews in Mandarin, Cantonese, or English, depending on interviewee preferences. Xin also oversaw recruitment, along with the translation and coding of the interview data. Edith Ngene Kambere, a Canadian graduate student and former settlement worker who originally migrated from Uganda, worked with Gillian. Edith ran the pilot study, collaborated in project design, interviewed African women, and transcribed all the interviews. Another research assistant, Mambo Masinda, a settlement worker originally from Congo, with a PhD from a Canadian university, interviewed African men. The multiplicity of languages, and commonality of English among participants who migrated from Africa, made English the only feasible interview language for diverse African immigrants, although levels of fluency varied.

The composition of the research teams was critical to the success of the two projects but did not solve the difficulties of researching across differences. No matter how committed we might be to working collaboratively as research teams, the principal investigators retained considerably more power in shaping the research agenda, processes, analysis, and communication of findings than did the research assistants, thus reproducing racialized and class-based power relations within the research teams themselves. Moreover, by virtue of being academic researchers, graduate students, and/or community-based researchers, the PIs and RAs had very different social locations than the research participants, most of whom were fairly marginal in terms of social class positions within Canada. In addition, the research was undertaken within the institutional context of tri-council funding guidelines (both projects were funded by the Social Science and Humanities

Research Council of Canada) and interpreted through university-based research ethics boards. The concerns circulating in feminist (and other) academic literatures, funding bodies, and university research ethics boards do not always mesh well with community concerns, yet they play a dominant role in shaping the research.

We followed a number of methodological strategies to situate individual interviews within broader community concerns and to more clearly hear what research participants told us about their experiences. These strategies included pilot studies to identify community-defined issues, consultation with key community experts, choice of language during interviews (in the study with Chinese immigrants), and interviewers who could identify at least to some degree as members of the community. We also held periodic debriefings about the research process, provided grocery vouchers and honoraria to cover child care and transportation, asked open-ended interview questions, engaged in iterative processes of grounded qualitative analysis, and strove to centre the voices of participants through the extensive use of quotations. In addition, a deliberate feminist participatory action research component (Frisby, Maguire, and Reid 2009) was built into the study with Chinese immigrants, as some of the women participated in a workshop and provided recommendations for policy change (with the assistance of translators) to forty policy makers. Such strategies have mitigated the worst excesses of masculinist, Eurocentric, and positivistic social research, but our respective research projects still raise important issues about the limitations of conducting feminist community research that traverses differences in race, language, and culture.

What follows is a series of reflections organized under three themes: first, we consider the dilemmas of defining *community* and acknowledging community diversity, while elucidating general processes that tend towards homogenization. Second, we discuss the complex issues raised about language, translation, and power through illustrative examples. Finally, we consider the difficulties embedded in representation, interpretation, and meaning making when we conduct research across difference.

Community, Diversity, and Homogenization

A key difficulty in any community-based research is to identity the community in question. This process can be as much an artifact of researchers' conceptualizations as self-defined social entities. Moreover, every community is internally diverse, so issues of whose views represent community concerns, practices, or experiences are also fraught with difficulties. In the context of research with communities that are marginalized in the larger society, as are immigrants of colour in the Canadian context, researchers face the additional danger of reinforcing stereotypes, Othering, or otherwise homogenizing and disempowering community members (Mohanty 2003). As feminist researchers, we want to disrupt homogenization, give voice to diversity, and empower participants in our research. Yet, these aims can be undermined by the very terms we use to describe the communities with which we work and the search for general themes to make sense of the data.

Both the African immigrant and Chinese immigrant communities exist in some material sense. In the 2006 Census, 27,260 people in Greater Vancouver identified their place of birth as a country in Africa (Statistics Canada 2006). However, fewer fall within the meaningful definition of African community emerging in the local context: those from sub-Saharan African countries who are racialized as black.[2] This smaller African community constitutes about 1 percent of the population in Metropolitan Vancouver (Statistics Canada 2006).[3] In contrast to the small African community, the Chinese community has a dominant presence in Vancouver. In the 2006 Census, 381,500 Vancouver residents – or one in every five people – identified their ethnicity as Chinese, and more than one-quarter of these residents were born abroad, mostly in China, Hong Kong, Taiwan, and Vietnam (Statistics Canada 2008, 32-33).

Both the African and Chinese immigrant communities are extremely diverse groups, and processes that lump each together as homogeneous categories reflect a larger context in which these differences are of little importance to dominant members of society. Hence, we need to problematize these terms as discursive forms of homogenization and silencing, and interrogate, rather than take for granted, whether these communities are, or are not, subjectively meaningful to those so defined. We also need to question whether our use of these categories for defining our research participants and projects perpetuates silencing or also has the potential to disrupt and unpack larger processes of marginalization.

Defining *community* is always complex and often contested, as the example of the local African community in Greater Vancouver illustrates. Edith, along with other self-identified members of the African community, has been working with Gillian on research with diverse black immigrants from sub-Saharan Africa since 2003 (see Creese and Kambere 2003; Creese 2007; Creese and Wiebe 2009). Part of our research involves asking how people identify themselves and what terms they find meaningful in the context of resettlement in Greater Vancouver. These terms of self-identification are often situational, depending on the context and the interlocutor. Many participants will identify by their national origin when speaking to another member of the larger African community, but almost all identify as African when speaking to someone perceived to be outside of that community. The point here is that the question, "Where are you from?" means something quite different depending on who asks.

In the context of generalized ignorance about Africa among many Canadians, and prevailing discourses that lump African countries together, the majority of the participants told us that in Vancouver they identify themselves first as African immigrants, and only secondarily by their national or sub-national (linguistic/ethnic) origin. Indeed, our research documents the emergence of a diasporic pan-African identity, linked not only to external pressures of Othering and marginalization, but also to the very small size of each national population in Greater Vancouver that draws people together across cleavages more likely to persist in contexts of larger populations.[4] Thus, the very small number of sub-Saharan Africans in the Vancouver area means that connections and community are developing across national and linguistic origins, with English the dominant language of communication within the African community. As a result, the term *African community* is a common – although not singular – form of self-identification that we also adopted in our research (Creese 2007).

In adopting this term, however, we also pave over very real differences among those from sub-Saharan Africa and contribute to homogenizing processes of marginalization. We help to make invisible the twenty-one different countries – with diverse languages, histories, and cultures – from which participants originated, thereby silencing the voices of those who resisted a generic African designation and ignoring the historical and ongoing conflicts within Africa that sometimes make common identification extremely difficult. Thus, we help to perpetuate colonizing processes through the myth that we don't need to account for these differences and complexities of diverse societies because black migrants from sub-Saharan Africa are essentially all the same.

At the same time, who comes to represent diverse African immigrants in our research also furthers these processes of silencing. Although participants came from twenty-one different countries, two-thirds came from only seven countries (Burundi, Democratic Republic of Congo, Ghana, Kenya,

Nigeria, Uganda, and Zimbabwe), in contrast to one or two participants each from fourteen other countries (Cape Verde Island, Congo-Brazzaville, Ethiopia, Guinea-Conakry, Malawi, Mozambique, Rwanda, Senegal, Sierra Leone, South Africa, Sudan, Swaziland, Togo, and Zambia), and none from over thirty other countries in Africa. Hence, some voices are amplified and overdetermine the research data and, ultimately, our understandings of the concerns of the "African community" now living in a large Canadian urban area. In our research, it was the voices of those from Commonwealth countries that were overrepresented, and this, too, shapes our understandings of definitions of community and identity. Conducting all the interviews in English clearly contributed to the dominance of voices from Commonwealth countries.

Diversity among Chinese women originating from Hong Kong, Taiwan, and various regions of China, in the second project, was also made invisible by conceptualizing these migrants through a common Chinese ethnicity, in spite of differences in how languages and cultural forms are shaped and re-shaped through divergent social geographies, political histories, and personal circumstances. In both cases, racialized notions of community can only be sustained from outside. In the case of immigrants from Africa, we have also suggested that the local social geography helps create connections across differences that are, indeed, giving rise to a new diasporic pan-African identity. For various Chinese immigrants, however, the size of the populations and the institutional depth of services, stores, businesses, and patterns of residential concentration catering to various Chinese diasporas, as well as multi-generational and intermarried Chinese Canadians, produce a rich tapestry of identities and linkages that cannot be seen as constituting an emerging single community.

The goal of the project with the immigrant Chinese women was to understand the role of physical activity programs offered in community centres (that are funded and operated by the City of Vancouver) in settlement. This project included only recent immigrants (one to ten years), and women originating from Mainland China (72 percent of participants) were overrepresented as interviewees, with an additional 12 percent originating from Hong Kong and 16 percent from Taiwan. Each of these geographical areas has different histories and linguistic and cultural traditions. The women also varied in age, with 77 percent of participants being between thirty-one and fifty years of age, 16 percent were thirty years and under, and 7 percent were over age fifty. Age certainly shaped different experiences and understandings of community centre programs. Economic status also varied, as 38 percent of the Chinese immigrant women reported annual household incomes of less than $20,000, 46 percent lived on $20,000-$50,000, with the remaining 12 percent reporting annual household incomes of over $50,000. As community centres in Canada are increasingly charging fees for physical activity programs, which is the result of the infiltration of neoliberal practices in local government (Frisby, Reid, and Ponic 2007), and as few residents, especially immigrants, are aware of the problematic subsidy policies (Taylor and Frisby 2010), inequitable access to services that could ease the difficulties associated with settlement is reinforced (Reid, Frisby, and Ponic 2002). Political histories and tensions tied to homeland geographies, together with linguistic, cultural, and generational effects, as well as social class, represent just some of the ways in which the Chinese immigrant women differed, whereas labelling them as one community for ease of description (as we have done in the title of this chapter) homogenizes them. Their marital status, the number of their children and dependants, and self-reported health status further reflected the diversity among them, all of which created different trajectories, coping strategies, and challenges for them upon arriving in Vancouver. Women with children were much more likely to hear about community centre programs through schools, while those who lived alone, were elderly, or had health problems were much less likely to know about or get involved in the physical activities provided.

In many ways, reference to the Chinese immigrant community is akin to the European immigrant community, a conceptual term almost never heard except when comparing trends among visible and non-visible minority immigrants.[5] Even with the formation of the European community as a political entity, the diversity of European countries and cultures is always acknowledged in Canada, while Chinese ethnicity overdetermines perceptions of a universal Chineseness, long after the demise of overtly racist discourses embedded in Canadian nation building (Mackey 2002; Thobani 2007). The very act of identifying interviewees as immigrants is double-edged: it brings attention to their circumstances of migration but, at the same time, signifies that they are "not from here," thus reifying processes of Othering. Stressing immigrant status can unintentionally feed into discourses of cultural assimilation, rather than positioning cultural diversity as an asset that contributes to the richness of Canadian society (Graham and Phillips 2007). For some, immigrants are just supposed to fit in and should not be a drain on social services. This makes feminist community research all the more important as a way of dismantling dominant discourses that marginalize those migrating from other countries and makes it crucial to carefully guard against the colonizing processes inherent in such discourses.

The terms we use for research purposes shape how we interpret our data, and have the potential to perpetuate discursive forms of Othering, as we seek to make sense of our findings. In both research projects, analyses of data involved transcribing the interviews; in the study on Chinese immigrant women, interviews were also translated into English; and in both studies, interview transcripts were coded using computer software for qualitative data analysis to help us identify patterns in the data.[6] Making sense of our data on African immigrants and Chinese women immigrants already presupposes appropriate categories of research design, coding, and analysis that direct us towards coherent narratives within the community. Strategies of generating codes from the data and listening hard for minority positions do not always disrupt homogenizing frameworks that are often desired by policy makers wanting to make generalizations from immigration research.

The main themes emerging from feminist research with marginalized communities typically highlight intersecting dimensions of inequality and form part of a larger transformative research agenda. Themes of hardship, poverty, racism, sexism, exclusion, and ongoing struggles to remake home in a new context are interwoven throughout both studies of immigrant experiences in ways that can also be read as pathologizing already marginalized groups. Finding the balance between documenting processes of marginalization to inform social change and highlighting forms of agency, resistance, and empowerment is always a difficult task. To downplay structural processes of marginalization supports neo-liberal narratives of individual responsibility and meritocracy; while underemphasizing agency can perpetuate discursive forms of violence, whereby immigrants are victims and social problems, thereby stabilizing common stereotypes even as we try to disrupt them.

The issue of whose agency and whose voices are profiled is also critical since communities are never homogeneous, and interpreting them from Western cultural frameworks is highly problematic. For example, in the African immigrant project the common experience of downward occupational mobility, low-wage employment, and isolated nuclear-family forms in Canada intensified domestic work and produced shifting gendered practices and expectations that saw wives/mothers demand more involvement of fathers/husbands in child care and other domestic duties. The pressures to redefine masculinity in a Canadian context in which men's authority in the household, civil society, and the economy was significantly undermined were, not surprisingly, resisted by many (though not all) men and were also resisted by some of the women interviewed. At the same time, we are acutely aware that illuminating the gendered impact of settlement processes and pressures in reconfiguring gender relations can easily be reinterpreted as yet another narrative of how Africans are more patriarchal and less progressive than Canadians. Moreover, from within the African community, we might be accused of giving more credence to women's views than to men's, a charge that has some weight and scholarly justification for research embedded in feminist theories and methodologies.

Similarly, in the Chinese immigration project, many of the women desired access to the physical activity programs offered by the twenty-two community centres in Vancouver for their children rather than for themselves. This solidifies stereotypes that immigrant women are not interested in such activities, further suggesting that the masculinist, individualistic, Eurocentric, and youth-oriented physical activity programs offered in Canada require no change (Frisby, Alexander, and Taylor 2010). Yet, when alternative approaches to recreation program development and delivery were imagined over the course of the interviews, several possible benefits of participation were identified, including reduced social isolation, improved physical and mental health, and opportunities to learn about activities in their new country. However, the principal investigator had never been to Mainland China, Hong Kong, or Taiwan, where the interviewees were from, and there is little literature available on how physical activity and recreation programs are offered in these countries. As a result, the interviewees and the research assistants had an essential role to play in educating the PI to reduce exclusions and misinterpretations based on her white, middle-class, Western understandings of community centre policies and program delivery practices and how they might assist or exclude immigrant women and their families. Negotiating this terrain is difficult enough for researchers who are from the community in question, but is even more fraught when researching across differences, facilities with languages, and other power relations shaping our processes of making meaning from research data.

Language, Translation, and Power

Research with African immigrants and Chinese immigrant women is complicated by language. The dominance of English-speaking researchers (outside Quebec) and the lack of racial, ethnic, and language diversity among faculty in Canadian post-secondary education means that fewer academic researchers communicate directly with immigrants in their mother tongues. This makes it more difficult to include immigrant communities in knowledge-production and policy-making processes.[7]

In both studies discussed in this chapter, the principal investigators were unilingual English speakers, yet they were largely responsible for the research design, analysis, and communication of the results. Research projects with African and Chinese immigrants were possible largely because of the other human resources available at the university and in the wider community. Graduate student research assistants came from Mainland China, Taiwan, and Uganda, and a community-based researcher (with a Canadian PhD but who had not found an academic job) came from Congo. All of these research assistants working on the two projects were multilingual. In addition, community partners working with African and Chinese immigrants helped to facilitate the research (e.g., SUCCESS, MOSAIC, Multicultural Family Services, Immigrant Services Society, and City of Vancouver community centres).

In the study with Chinese immigrant women, the ability of participants to voice their issues and concerns was enhanced by speaking in their mother tongue to another person who had also migrated to Canada. For instance, one participant told us:

> Things have been accumulating in my heart for a long time, and I need to speak to somebody who will listen.

The ability to express herself in her mother tongue helped her to feel less isolated. At the same time, language issues were complicated because the interviews, transcriptions, and translations were often done in other languages and/or from different cultural, racialized, and classed positions.

Chinese as a language is not singular, as it comprises different dialects and written forms in diverse spaces.[8] For example, English was the sole official language of Hong Kong from 1843 to 1974, and Chinese became another official language only in 1974. The majority of people in Hong Kong did not speak Mandarin, but some started to learn it before the handover of Hong Kong to the People's Republic of China in 1997. Since then, English and Chinese have been the constitutionally defined official languages under the Basic Law of Hong Kong and the Official Languages Ordinance. In practice, the official languages in Hong Kong are *liangwen sanyu*, which means two written languages (English and Chinese) and three spoken languages (English, Mandarin, and Cantonese). While traditional Chinese is written in

Hong Kong and Taiwan, a simplified version is the official written language in Mainland China. Mandarin is mostly spoken and the official spoken language in Mainland China and Taiwan, while Cantonese is officially spoken in Hong Kong and in some parts of China as a local dialect.

This leads to a politics of language within the often-assumed homogeneous Chinese-speaking community. Issues emerged in the interviews regarding different levels of communication, comprehension, relationships, and dynamics with the researchers. Additionally, issues arose in terms of expressions and representability between those who spoke in their mother tongues (e.g., some interviewees), those who used their second language/dialect (e.g., some interviewees and the research assistants), and those who are interpreting and writing about the data in the dominant colonial English language (e.g., the RAs and the PI). An example of the complexities involved occurred when Xin prepared documents to undergo ethics approval for research on human subjects prior to recruiting interviewees. She first drafted the research procedures and documents in English, which were reviewed with Wendy, and then translated the documents into Chinese. As a recent immigrant from Mainland China, Xin speaks the official oral language, Mandarin, and writes in simplified Chinese, the official written form. When she contacted the settlement service agency SUCCESS[9] to recruit interviewees, she realized that to reach Chinese immigrant women from Taiwan and Hong Kong, she needed to convert the documents into traditional Chinese and use vocabularies comprehensible to Cantonese speakers. To reduce confusion and misinterpretation and to encourage participation in the research project across diverse Chinese dialects, recruitment posters and documents were prepared in traditional and simplified Chinese. Amendments were then submitted to the research ethics board with the new translations, although it is unlikely that ethics board reviewers could read the amendments in all of these dialects.

The language ability of the principal investigator and the research assistants made English, Mandarin, and simplified Chinese the default languages in the project design and marginalized other Chinese language forms and dialects. During the interview process, since all three Chinese research assistants spoke Mandarin but not Cantonese, Mandarin speakers, who were mostly from Mainland China and Taiwan, were in a more advantaged position, and they experienced smoother and more direct communication with the interviewers.[10] Cantonese speakers from Hong Kong had to undergo a linguistic adaptation to articulate their responses to interview questions, speaking either in Mandarin or in English, which was possible in the case of some young and well-educated women, or speak through an interpreter hired from the immigrant service agency SUCCESS. The issues of translation compounded the layers of possible misinterpretation for Cantonese speakers. Employing linguistic adaptation was also experienced by some participants from Mainland China, especially those from southern regions, who speak their own dialects at home. For them, Mandarin is not their mother tongue or everyday language, and it is often only spoken at school and on official or professional occasions.

Speaking Mainland Mandarin also means using certain terms and expressions charged with official ideologies, as embedded in a specific political history as the official spoken language of the People's Republic of China. For example, there are several Chinese terms that can be used to refer to "doing physical activities," such as *zuoyudong* (doing exercise or doing sports), *duanlian shenti* (tempering or steeling the body), *jianshen* (strengthening the body), and *huodong shenti* (warming up the body). Many participants from Mainland China often use the official term *duanlian* to refer to doing physical exercise or "to work out." Yet, *duanlian* is a term that frequently appeared in Mao-era slogans encouraging people to prepare their bodies for the revolution and the building of the socialist nation (Brownell 1995). As Tina Mai Chen points out, the term *duanlian* points to the purpose of the exercise: to forge a proletarian iron body for Maoist China to embody China's future. People were encouraged to build up a good physique to defend the country (*duanlian shenti baowei zuguo*), build a good physique for socialism (*weile shehuizhuyi jiji duanlian shenti*), and temper oneself through manual labour (*laodong duanlian*) (Chen 2003, 365). *Duanlian* was also used to refer to the sending of intellectuals and urban youth to the factories and the countryside to be re-educated by workers and peasants, as a reform initiative through physical labour. *Duanlian* also has a gendered dimension. In stories about the socialist female model workers or the iron girls of the Mao era (Chen 2003; Jin 2006), these women had to *duanlian* or reform their physical bodies as well as redefine femininity when they moved into traditionally male areas of work. The use of the term *duanlian*, thus, does not only mean "to work out" in the Western sense, but evokes other historically and politically charged connotations, which link the exercise of the individual body to the creation of the proletarian workers' body and the building of the Chinese socialist state.

The connections between language use, ethnicity, and cultural values mean that what is suppressed by the imposition of standard Chinese is not only the plurality of dialects, but also alternative ways of experiencing, interpreting, and representing experience. As Kwai-Chung Lo (2000) has argued, by unifying the tools of exchange and communication and creating hierarchies of one dialect over another, the hegemonic Mandarin production of meaning often eliminates deviant voices that emerge in other Chinese dialects and is, therefore, associated with cultural assimilation. For people who speak dialects, especially for those from Hong Kong, using Mandarin is often associated with subjection and reformations of subjectivity (Lo 2000). Furthermore, as Rey Chow (2000) points out, Mandarin is also the white men's Chinese language that becomes the default in research on China overseas. As a result, the use of Mandarin in the research project on Chinese immigrant women may remind some women of their position of being inferior in the dominant culture both at home and abroad, thereby limiting their narrative agency.

In the study of African immigrants, issues of language and power are directly rooted in centuries of European colonialism, with the language of former colonial powers constituting at least one of the official languages of most African countries. Language was an instrument of colonial power (Willinsky 1998), and the subjugation of indigenous languages was a key part of the colonial process (Phillipson and Skutnabb-Kangas 1995; Pennycock 1998). In post-colonial contexts, fluency in the official European language (e.g., English in the Commonwealth and French in *la francophonie*) remains simultaneously a mark of class advantage within African countries (i.e., evidence of attaining high school or post-secondary education) and evidence of an inferior version of the language, as contained in different accents on a global scale from the dominant vantage points of former European powers and their white settler colonies (Lippi-Green 1997; Bourdieu 1977). Indeed, one of the key themes to emerge from the research with women and men who migrated from sub-Saharan Africa is the pervasive and multiple forms of discrimination facing those who speak with African English accents (Creese and Kambere 2003; Creese 2007, 2010). Yet, this same stigmatized language/accent was the only medium that could be used to explore the terms of linguistic and other forms of marginalization and agency in Canada.

Participants were drawn from twenty-one different countries in sub-Saharan Africa and spoke dozens of different languages and dialects, the vast majority of which were unknown to the multilingual research assistants, and all were unknown to the principal investigator. Three-quarters of participants were fluent in English, and one-quarter were fluent in French before migration to Canada. However, only one RA was fluent in French, while both RAs and the PI were fluent in English. For those who were not fluent in English before they came to Canada, difficulties of communication and translation were that much greater. Language issues compounded the inequalities of social class (i.e., with less affluent migrants being less likely to be schooled in English in their countries of origin), gender (i.e., with more men than women possessing higher levels of education), and geopolitics (i.e., with those coming from Commonwealth Africa more likely to be trained in English).

The difficulties in translation can lead to misunderstandings and mis-interpretations, and what is lost in translation makes certain experiences unrepresentable. For instance, the term *physical activities* does not have an equivalent in different Chinese dialects. To make it comprehensible for Chinese participants, the RAs had to use Chinese terms such as *zuoyundon* (doing sports) and *duanlian* (doing exercise). This not only affects com-munication and comprehension between participants, RAs, and PIs, it also plays an important role in the representation and interpretation of these experiences and is, hence, critical to the enterprise of meaning making.

In feminist participatory action research, translation and interpretation are important in facilitating participation, mutual understanding, and ex-change between members of an ethnocultural community and the English-speaking researchers, policy makers, and community service providers. For instance, in the project with Chinese immigrant women, we invited research participants to a Multiculturalism and Physical Activity Workshop to share research findings and discuss policy initiatives. Five of the Chinese immi-grant women who were interviewed agreed to share their experiences and join the discussions, and some policy makers told us that this was their first opportunity to listen directly to immigrants. By learning more about every-day life experiences of the women, and listening to their articulate and thoughtful comments, workshop participants from local, provincial, and federal governments indicated that they were inspired to think from differ-ent perspectives other than their own, and view the women not as needy victims but as active agents in shaping policy alternatives. For many English-speaking participants in the workshop, this was also a mutual learning process on how to engage in cross-language and cross-cultural communica-tion with the assistance of the multilingual RAs and a hired interpreter from SUCCESS. The policy makers slowed down their conversation and listened patiently to panel discussions being translated from languages that they did not understand, giving them a momentary glimpse of how differences in language limit participation in community. Chinese immigrant women, on the other hand, became more aware of the value of their participation, and all of them said that they gained a sense of empowerment as the workshop progressed, even though they admitted to being very nervous at the outset of their panel presentation. A main limitation of the workshop was that the five panel members did not represent the views of all fifty women who were interviewed, nor of the many other Chinese immigrant women who did not participate in the study. Nonetheless, the workshop was successful as an initial step in bridging the disconnections that existed between policy makers, researchers, and immigrants. The actions emanating from the workshop are now being tracked to determine if policy change in the area of multiculturalism and physical activity will occur.

Interpretation and the Politics of Meaning Making

The use of English as the primary research language conveys a Canadian conception and academic framing of issues, and in the case of our studies, facilitates a feminist agenda. This is evident in the conceptual language that frames our research designs, as well as specific research questions addressed. Yet, such framing can close down rather than open up productive dialogues around key issues. In the study of African immigrants, changing circumstances leading to challenging definitions of masculinity were troubling for many men and for some women too. Feminist ways of thinking about changing gender relations in the context of downward mobility in the labour market, two-income families, the loss of extended family help, lack of child care, isolated nuclear families in Canada, and different expectations around parenting and schooling were helpful for thinking through patterns in the research. But these same frameworks were rejected by some participants for whom challenges to masculinity were the product of a loss of tradition, culture, and respect for authority. Questions rooted in feminist understandings that did not engage fully with notions of tradition and culture tended to close off the latter lines of inquiry.

On the other hand, interview questions informed by feminist theory can help to bring issues and concerns to participants' attention and encourage them to interpret and frame their understandings of certain events in different ways. For example, in the project with Chinese immigrant women, an interview question about the Olympic and Paralympic Winter Games held in Vancouver in 2010 opened up discussion based on the feminist analysis that it is largely male business and political elites who benefit from the hosting of such mega events (Lenskyj 2008). Given that considerable resources are diverted away from community physical activity programs and social services to host mega-sporting events, this introduced a feminist people-centred, citizens' rights-based response from several interviewees that could inform policy makers about redistributions of physical activity investments. Inspired by these interview questions, some women started to make connections between the Olympics and their everyday lives, commenting on the tangible personal benefits (e.g., being inspired to become more physically active and learn about new sports done in Canada) and the significant disadvantages, such as the individual and collective costs of hosting the Games (e.g., higher taxes and housing costs, increased transportation problems, a lack of access to legacy facilities). In their responses, some immigrant women acknowledged that physical activity programs in Canada are directed more at children, especially their sons, illustrating their observations of the ageist and gendered ways in which programs are delivered. They provided numerous suggestions on how Olympic organizers could include them (e.g., by giving tours of facilities and instruction in winter sports), and they felt they would be assets as volunteers who could assist Chinese-speaking visitors coming to the event. Representatives from Legacies Now, an organization associated with the Vancouver 2010 Winter Olympic Games charged with promoting social inclusion, were in attendance at the Multiculturalism and Physical Activity Workshop, and they heard directly from the women about this topic, thereby including them more directly in the politics of meaning making. Whether this will translate into greater inclusion remains to be seen, as mega-events like the Olympics have a long history of problems, exclusions, and broken promises (Lenskyj 2008).

Another aspect of the politics of meaning making involves providing opportunities for community members to interpret, respond to, or contest meanings emerging from the research. For example, findings from the African immigrant project have been presented at two different community forums, venues that can provide reciprocal conversations about meaning. It remains the case, however, that community members largely respond to narratives defined without their input.

Conclusion

This chapter highlights some of the difficulties of conducting feminist community research across racial, language, and cultural differences, and yet we remain committed to this type of research as one way of illuminating the voices of immigrants to contribute to a social justice agenda. By describing our research experiences from a critical stance, we hope to encourage improved methodologies that further unpack the inherent power imbalances and intricacies involved. At the same time, critical reflections such as these leave relations of power and privilege in representation intact while reminding us of the potential dangers of privileging certain voices and further marginalizing other ethnocultural immigrant communities, thereby reproducing or reinforcing inequalities among and across immigrant groups. It is important to acknowledge that many other ethnocultural communities are not currently receiving attention from researchers and research funders, creating significant gaps in whose voices are heard and potentially acted upon. In the long run, we hope to facilitate diverse forms of community-based research, develop more egalitarian community-academic engagements, and encourage more young people from a wide range of communities to engage in critical research methodologies.

NOTES

1 Frisby was born in Canada. Creese migrated from Britain at the age of two and was raised in Canada. Although she is technically an immigrant, the privileges associated with white Anglo dominance in Canada have never made her or her family "outsiders" in the sense in which most recent immigrants experience.

2 This excludes those who migrated from countries in sub-Saharan Africa but are racialized as white, Asian, or Arabic.

3 Less than 1 percent of the Greater Vancouver population (20,670 people out of just over 2 million residents) identified as black in the 2006 Census. This includes people of African descent who were born in Canada or migrated from other parts of the world, including the Caribbean, the United Kingdom, and the United States. Statistics Canada, 2006 Census, http://www12.statcan.ca/census-recensement/ 2006 (downloaded 13 January 2009).

4 The contrast between Vancouver and Toronto is especially marked in this regard. Toronto has much larger populations from specific African countries (particularly Ghana, Somalia, and Ethiopia) – in fact, there are as many Ghanaians in Toronto as there are sub-Saharan Africans in Vancouver. In the context of large populations from one country, national identities take precedence.

5 The terms *visible* and *non-visible minority* are labels used by the federal government that reinforce the dominance of "whiteness" through the association with "non-visible."

6 The African immigrant project used MAXqda software, and the Chinese immigrant women project used Atlas ti.

7 We are not suggesting that it is only university-based faculty who do research with immigrant groups, even though this is the focus of this chapter because of our locations within the academy. Community-based research occurs outside the university, and it may occur in multiple languages.

8 *Chinese* is an umbrella term for different forms of written and spoken Chinese languages. There are two standard sets of Chinese characters for spoken Chinese.

Speakers of different dialects of Chinese have historically used one single formal written language. The contemporary Chinese written language is based on the grammar and vocabulary of Mandarin. Many grammatical/lexical deviations in dialects other than Mandarin are regarded as "slang" (literally, "vulgar language"). These varieties are distinct in their spoken forms only, and when written, are common across the country. Therefore, even though China is home to hundreds of relatively unique spoken languages, literate people are usually able to communicate through written language.

9 SUCCESS is an immigrant settlement agency that the majority of Chinese immigrants in Vancouver go to for assistance with housing and employment upon arrival.

10 We asked our participants to indicate the languages they speak at home, which can be considered the languages they feel most comfortable with. Among the fifty participants, sixteen of them speak Cantonese, two speak other dialects, and twenty-five speak Mandarin at home. Five participants speak both Mandarin and another dialect, and two speak a mixture of Mandarin and English at home.

REFERENCES

Bourdieu, Pierre. 1977. "The Economics of Linguistic Exchanges." *Social Science Information* 16(6): 645-68.

Brownell, Susan. 1995. *Training the Body for China: Sports in the Moral Order of the People's Republic.* Chicago: University of Chicago Press.

Chen, Tina Mai. 2003. "Proletarian White and Working Bodies in Mao's China." *Positions: East Asia Cultures Critique* 11(2): 361-93.

Chow, Rey. 2000. Introduction. In R. Chow, ed., *Modern Chinese Literary and Cultural Studies in the Age of Theory*, 1-25. Durham and London: Duke University Press.

Creese, Gillian. 2007. "From Africa to Canada: Bordered Spaces, Border Crossings and Imagined Communities." In V. Agnew, ed., *Interrogating Race and Racism*, 456-502. Toronto: University of Toronto Press.

–. 2010. "Erasing English Language Competency: African Migrants in Vancouver, Canada." *Journal of International Migration and Integration* 11(3): 295-313.

Creese, Gillian, and Edith Ngene Kambere. 2003. "'What Colour Is Your English?'" *Canadian Review of Sociology and Anthropology* 50(5): 565-73.

Creese, Gillian, and Brandy Wiebe. 2009. "'Survival Employment': Gender and Deskilling among African Immigrants in Canada." *International Migration.* doi: /0.1111/j.1468-2435.2009.00531.x.

Frisby, Wendy, Ted Alexander, and Janna Taylor. 2010. "Play Is Not a Frill: Poor Youth Facing the Past, Present, and Future of Public Recreation in Canada." In Mona Gleason, Tamara Myers, Lesley Paris, and Veronica Strong-Boag, eds., *Lost Kids: Vulnerable Children and Youth in Twentieth-Century Canada and the United States*, 215-29. Vancouver: UBC Press.

Frisby, Wendy, Patricia Maguire, and Colleen Reid. 2009. "The 'F' Word Has Everything to Do with It: How Feminist Theories Inform Action Research." *Action Research* 7(1): 13-19.

Frisby, Wendy, Colleen Reid, and Pamela Ponic. 2007. "Levelling the Playing Field: Promoting the Health of Poor Women through a Community Development Approach to Recreation." In Kevin Young and Phillip White, eds., *Sport and Gender in Canada*, 121-36. Don Mills, ON: Oxford University Press.

Graham, Katherine, and Susan D. Phillips. 2007. "Another Fine Balance: Managing Diversity in Canadian Cities." In Keith Banting, Thomas J. Courchene, and Leslie Seidle, eds., *The Art of the State: Belonging? Diversity, Recognition and Shared Citizenship in Canada*, 155-94. Montreal: Institute for Research on Public Policy.

Jin, Yihong. 2006. "Rethinkng the 'Iron Girls': Gender and Labour during the Chinese Cultural Revolution." *Gender and History* 18(3): 613-34.

Lenskyj, Helen Jefferson. 2008. *Olympic Industry Resistance: Challenging Olympic Power and Propaganda*. New York: SUNY Press.

Lippi-Green, Rosina. 1997. *English with an Accent: Language, Ideology and Discrimination in the United States*. New York: Routledge.

Lo, Kwai-Chung. 2000. "Look Who's Talking: The Politics of Orality in Transitional Hong Kong Mass Culture." In Rey Chow, ed., *Modern Chinese Literary and Cultural Studies in the Age of Theory*, 181-98. Durham and London: Duke University Press.

Mackey, Eva. 2002. *The House of Difference: Cultural Politics and National Identity in Canada*. Toronto: University of Toronto Press.

Mohanty, Chandra Talpate. 2003. "Under Western Eyes: Feminist Scholarship and Colonial Discourses." In Reina Lewis and Sara Mills, eds., *Feminist Postcolonial Theory: A Reader*, 49-74. Edinburgh: Edinburgh University Press.

Pennycook, Alastair. 1998. *English and the Discourses of Colonialism*. London: Routledge.

Phillipson, Robert, and Tove Skutnabb-Kangas. 1995. "Language Rights in Post-Colonial Africa." In Tove Skutnabb-Kangas and Robert Phillipson, eds., *Linguistic Human Rights: Overcoming Linguistic Discrimination*, 335-46. Berlin: Mouton de Gruyter.

Reid, Colleen, Wendy Frisby, and Pamela Ponic. 2002. "Confronting Two-Tiered Community Recreation and Poor Women's Exclusion: Promoting Inclusion, Health, and Social Justice. *Canadian Women's Studies* 21(3): 88-94.

Statistics Canada. 2006. http://www12.statcan.ca/census-recensement/2006; and http://www12.statcan.ca/census06/data/profiles/sip/RetrieveProduct Table (down-loaded 13 Jan. 2009).

–. 2008. *Canada's Ethnocultural Mosaic, 2006 Census*. April 2008. Catalogue no. 97-562-X. Ottawa: Statistics Canada.

Taylor, Janna, and Wendy Frisby. 2010. "Addressing Inadequate Leisure Access Policies through Citizen Engagement." In Heather Mair, Susan M. Arai, and Donald G. Reid, eds., *Decentering Work: Critical Perspectives on Leisure, Social Policy, and Human Development*, 30-45. Calgary: University of Calgary Press.

Thobani, Sunera. 2007. *Exalted Subjects: Studies in the Making of Race and Nation in Canada*. Toronto: University of Toronto Press.

Twine, France Windance. 2000. "Racial Ideologies and Racial Methodologies." In
    F.W. Twine and J. Warren, eds., *Racing Research, Researching Race:
    Methodological Dilemmas in Critical Race Studies,* 1-34. New York: New York
    University Press.
Willinsky, John. 1998. *Learning to Divide the World: Education at Empire's End.*
    Minneapolis: University of Minnesota Press.

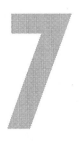

Tangled Nets and Gentle Nettles
Negotiating Research Questions with Immigrant Service Organizations

TARA GIBB AND EVELYN HAMDON

In Canada, the integration of immigrants into the labour force has for some years been a federal priority in funding both programs and research. Some new immigrants are perceived to have "weak capital" – to lack certain "essential skills" that will ensure employment (HRDC 2002) – and federal research is intended to determine clear solutions to this perceived problem. Immigrant service organizations (ISOs) are important partners in a relationship that the literature portrays as complex at best. Empirical studies have shown the relation of state and immigrant service organizations to be mutually dependent with shared goals (Holder 1998), but also potentially subjugating, turning ethnic organizations into extensions of state-coordinated activities and instruments of social control (Feldman 2002; Ng 1996). Those taking a more benign view maintain that immigrant service organizations act as social service providers to maintain ethnic identities and promote integration (Guo 2002). Further, argue Beyene et al. (1996), organizations (such as ISOs) are active politically in combatting racism in social services. University-based researchers have inserted their questions into the mix, amplifying critical concerns related to cross-cultural identity, language, and power relations involved in the process of immigrant "settlement." Working with immigrant organizations, academic researchers have joined the protest over issues such as deskilling and the decredentializing of qualifications (Henry et al. 2000; Mojab 1999; Reitz 2003), and the sexism combined with racism experienced by women immigrants, who often labour in exploitative conditions (Ng 1996; Gannage 1999).

This chapter explores the negotiations that determine what becomes "researched" within collaborative state-funded research frameworks related to new immigrants and employment. The discussion draws from our case studies of two community-based feminist immigrant service organizations and analyzes cultural influences on the shifting object of research and the positionalities of the actors (funders, researchers, clients, and organizational administrators and staff). While previous discussions have focused on the immigrant women's experiences with migration and struggles for recognition in Canada's employment systems (Gibb, Hamdon, and Jamal 2008; Gibb and Hamdon 2010), in this chapter we turn our attention to the relationships between researchers, agency administrators, and the state in negotiating research questions. We draw on Fraser's (1995, 2001) and Feldman's (2002) conceptualizations of recognition and redistribution to rethink our research relationships and to consider the possibilities for establishing more equitable approaches to conducting collaborative research with federal and community constituencies.

Struggle of Feminism in the Lingering "Shadow" of Masculine Positivism

We (university-based researchers) conducted case studies with two community organizations in Canada that provide educational and settlement services for new immigrant women, mostly visible minorities. These two case studies were part of a larger project involving four immigrant service organizations. Each case involved the observation of everyday routines within the organizations, selected classes, and meetings. Documents such as annual reports and informational materials prepared for clients were examined. Interviews were conducted with immigrant clients, volunteers, paid staff, and organizational administrators to understand their differing perspectives about what new immigrants learned through the organization's activities and that were most valuable in terms of finding employment. In addition, we asked what they needed most in order to become integrated into the labour force.

Both organizations were established in the 1980s and offer programs focused on employability, representing their work as supporting women's personal well-being as well as job-skill training. In total, twenty-one women were interviewed, including administrators, staff, volunteers, and clients. Twelve were current or former clients or learners, five were staff members, and two were members of the board (one from each ISO). Their respective

positions and relationships within each organization are complex. Some of
the volunteers were formers students, some of the staff had been both students and volunteers, and all but one of those interviewed were immigrant
women who had migrated to Canada from China, Hong Kong, Zimbabwe,
Pakistan, India, Japan, and Iran.

Two constituencies with contrasting research cultures were involved in
developing and funding the original research questions: Human Resources
and Development Canada (HRDC), accustomed to contracted research that
produces short-term results and policy-targeted findings; and the Social
Sciences and Humanities Research Council (SSHRC), the national social
science granting agency promoting scholarly inquiry with three- and five-
year timelines. The resulting federally funded and SSHRC-administered
"strategic" grant was awarded to successful proposals addressing the previously determined research question: *"How can the voluntary sector be an
effective instrument for delivering programmes for the acquisition of essential
skills to Canada's immigrant populations?"* The federal government is primarily concerned with increasing the integration of new immigrants into
the labour force. Partly because of perceptions that national productivity is
slipping, a skills shortage is looming, and immigrants are not finding employment as rapidly as they might because of their lack of employability
skills, including language facility, "working with people," "reading and writing documents," and the like, in the later 1990s, an "Essential Skills" (HRSDC
2004) initiative was developed by the Canadian government to measure and
promote development of nine essential skill areas identified as essential in
all occupations.

Preliminary reviews of the literature coupled with exploratory conversations with ISO staff resulted in our own research questions becoming increasingly focused on understanding how ISOs and their "clients"
conceptualized and developed the knowledge and identities that they believed would secure long-term, hopefully satisfying, employment for immigrant women. Further, we began to pay attention to the ways in which
staff and client observations amounted to critiques of current policies and
practices. In addition to this, the community organizations had their own
layers of research questions emerging from their everyday work with immigrant women: these related to practices of teaching/learning and grants-
manship, as well as broader issues of immigrants' skill recognition, subtle
racism in workplaces, and their external positioning relative to immediate
political issues (such as the Sharia law debate). Add to this the silencing of
their ability to engage in collective advocacy work, which was the result of

changes to federal funding guidelines, and what we quickly found was that women administrators in the community ISOs had learned to tread gently around the tangled nets of funding and conflicting research questions to ensure survival of their (often precarious) organizations and cultures (Scott 2003). They were aware of both their own importance to the federal agenda of improving immigrant integration and of being "handled" gingerly by funders who treated them like nettles: their feminist politics and convictions about structural racism were stinging irritants avoided by state funders. These ISO administrators clearly articulated to us the gulf between their own research needs – which included issues of institutionalized and systemic racism – and the questions posed and funded by external constituencies, including the academics and graduate students who were frequent interlopers in their organizations. As well, they indicated frustration because of their inability to move their research questions forward despite multiple forays into research partnerships, a situation they believe arises from the failure of governments and funders to value their analysis of immigration and settlement issues.

At the same time, the community ISOs drew upon linguistic and political strategies to configure their programs and knowledge needs in ways that could tap available government funds and grants. Sometimes this led to delivering programs that instructors knew neglected, and in the worst cases exacerbated, the problem of increasing new immigrants' employability, focusing individuals on superficial "life skills" delivered in short classroom programs. According to those we spoke with, these sorts of programs cannot address the issues of cultural knowledge and confidence that women clients said they needed to obtain employment. Further, such programming continued to sidestep complex systemic issues, which staff claimed were the most significant in determining immigrant women's ability to gain employment: racism, non-recognition of educational and professional designations, and North American language expectations (e.g., the focus on accent reduction).

Nested Relationships and Equity Issues

Negotiating relationships and research agendas can highlight disparities of power with and in collaborative research projects, disparities that often are the result of the absence of a common frame and language for negotiating research questions, purposes, and benefits with the partner organizations. The relational and political issues of collaboration led to individual reflection and collective discussion about our multiple and sometimes conflicting responsibilities. We struggled with the sociality of the relationships, wondering to what degree, as feminist researchers working within a traditional masculinist/positivist research environment, we were able or free to act upon the multiple points of connection (social, cultural, ethnic, political) that we had with the women with whom we were working in the ISOs. Our sense of responsibility to our community partners, and to individual participants, was differently constituted by our various subject positions as researchers, and influenced by our particular orientations to the community and the academy, our various senses of research protocol in general, and especially of this project.

In this section, we (two of the graduate research assistants) recount our reflections on our struggles as neophyte researchers learning the protocols of conducting research. In addition, we were learning to negotiate the responsibility of relationships and we felt the push and pull among senior faculty members, the community participants (administrators and clients), and civil servants representing funding bodies. At each community organization, one faculty member and one graduate research assistant worked closely with the staff and executive to determine the parameters for proceeding with the research. Senior faculty members demonstrated great confidence in our ability to conduct research, evidenced by the fact that early on they trusted us to make site visits on our own to gather data. They are women we respect as researchers and feminists; thus, we felt a strong responsibility to live up to their expectations, even if confidence in our own abilities was lacking. At the same time, we were also negotiating personal responsibilities to the administrators and staff of the immigrant service organizations.

Tara's Experience of the Research Relationships

I had had several years of experience working and living outside of Canada, in addition to several years of teaching in immigrant community programs in Canada. This was my first venture into academic research. I had returned to university to complete a master's degree because I wanted to make sense of the problematic issues that I had encountered in my working life. I had not been in a university setting for many years, and I was still unsure of my own intellectual capacities to do research. Nonetheless, being offered the opportunity to be mentored into the research culture was a long-hoped-for dream. I was particularly drawn to participating in this project because it involved an opportunity to think about and influence policy, an area I have long been interested in. I now realize how naive I was about the research process and its ability to influence policy. While attending two meetings involving community organization administrators, civil servants, faculty members, and graduate students, it became apparent that meeting participants came with conflicting expectations about what the research process would achieve. Some participants wanted the research to verify the viability of already existing programs; others saw the meetings as an advocacy opportunity; while some saw them as a chance to negotiate the divide between theoretical and policy debates. While participating in these meetings, I began to reflect upon the way in which a person's perceived status in a group influences the opportunities that he or she has to speak. Not all voices were equally heard or valued. I began to wonder to what extent we, our community partners and the research team, could contribute to transforming policy unless fundamental changes were made to the dynamic of power that flowed through the relationships.

Through the research process, I also became aware of the murky and ambiguous nature of doing research. In the early stages of the research, the original state-created research question, formulated by the funding agency, was presented to administrators. They began asking "sideways" questions about the federal funding policies: they wanted to know if Essential Skills was a new source for possible program grants. When we indicated our own interest in understanding immigrant women's experiences in learning what they needed in order to obtain meaningful employment, they approved the general tenor of the question but appeared to have little interest in the results. They began to negotiate obliquely, through stories and allusions, the direction in which they felt the research ought to go. To illustrate, at a community forum presenting research on immigrant elders, one senior board member pointedly drew me aside to discuss in detail her concerns about the research presented at this event being taken up from, in her words, "a neoliberal standpoint." A team from the same university had conducted the research, completely distinct from our project. I was unsure of what to make of this conversation. Was she trying to tell me indirectly that she hoped our research would take a different standpoint from this other research? Was she trying to suggest that our questions take a different form, that they weren't really addressing the issues important to the community? Alternatively, was she hoping we could have some influence on the political stance of this other research team, given that we shared an institutional affiliation? I wanted to be respectful of her concerns, but as a novice researcher, I was unsure of how to respond and unclear about what was expected of me. At times, I felt as if I was wandering through a forest with no sense of which direction was north.

Returning to the university from site visits to discuss observations and interviews with my research mentor, I felt a weight of expectation that I should be able to discuss with her "relevant" data, data that would help us "answer" the question. However, collecting "relevant" data was highly dependent on the state of relationships in the communities and our relationships with the communities. Site visits not only included observing classes and conducting interviews, but also attending community events. Sometimes it felt as if participants (administrators and employees) were suspicious of our intent and did not want to share information for fear of compromising their current jobs in the organization even though ethical mechanisms were in place to ensure anonymity. In other examples, occasionally during interviews, participants who were clients of the ISOs began to cry as they described the struggles and loneliness that they felt in migrating to Canada. I responded intuitively to their concerns, but later felt unsure if I had acted appropriately and began to question the ethics of asking women to talk about their experiences. Their struggles did not stem from a lack of "essential skills," but from a lack of recognition for the knowledge and skills that they already possessed. At other times, it seemed as if some members of the executive were disappointed to see me, the graduate student, and not my more experienced and influential research mentor. While my research mentor had faith in my abilities, I realized my student status did not carry the same social capital for ISO administrators as that of a full professor.

As we gradually gained entry and heard the stories of the women staff and clients of the organizations, we naturally began to alter, or subvert, our own academic line of inquiry. For example, instead of focusing on immigrant women's learning of skills related to employment, we realized that key issues lay in confidence, language perceptions, and employer reactions. Meanwhile, the organizational administrators were most interested in finding practical solutions to organizational problems and in generating data about issues in their communities that they felt needed attention (i.e., funding for programs they would deliver) from policy makers. In a true spirit of collaboration, we wondered to what extent we could alter our research focus even further to meet these research needs of the organizations.

Evelyn's Experience of the Research Relationships

Looking back, it appears to me that our relationships and our perspectives of what constituted responsibility and reciprocity were affected, at least in part, by our various positionalities and complicated by particular cultural and structural issues. Pre-existing relationships between and among some of the researchers and some of the community participants shaped emergent senses of responsibility, indebtedness, and reciprocity. For example, I shared a close cultural tie with the executive director of one of the ISOs, a tie that perhaps kindly disposed the executive director and other staff towards my presence as a researcher. And while this tie was helpful in establishing trust as an entry point, it also carried with it an implicit understanding that it ought to secure some sort of influence within the research relationship. If I was drawing upon past relationships (cultural, gendered, working, etc.) to help the research team gain access to an organization, it appeared to me that our feminist principles, regarding the mutuality of women's work and working relationships, necessitated our contributing something to the relationship. The process of negotiating this "something" brought into sharp relief our various understandings of responsibility and reciprocity.

For example, a request from Organization A for compensation for their time and resources (space for interviews, use of staff time, borrowing of materials for document analysis) sparked a dialogue within the research team about the efficacy, ethics, and equity of contributing to one site when we could not contribute to all, and raised questions about our own complex relations with the community and with the academy. In the absence of a clearly defined set of obligations, where did our primary responsibilities reside? As a student, I was acutely aware that I had little cultural capital to draw upon; however, my long-standing relationship (as a colleague) with my community research partners only served as a reminder that I had responsibilities to the community and to those relationships as well.

In addition, the questions regarding compensation for time and resources given in the research relationship highlighted (at least for me) what I viewed as our relative impoverishment with respect to what we could offer in return for the riches the staff and students of the ISO offered us. My own feelings were mixed. I felt kinship and friendship with the executive director of the ISO and was sympathetic to the organization's continual struggle for enough funds to continue to do its work. Yet, I also understood the ethical complications regarding the need for equal treatment of our community colleagues. It is somewhat simplistic to say that I felt torn between feelings of responsibility for my community-based colleagues and my responsibilities to be a careful novice scholar.

Negotiating a shared, or at least a tolerable, level of understanding of reciprocity led me to consider that there were other forms that it might take.

I hoped that we might offer a conduit for their voices while they provided us with data – the stuff of research. Perhaps we could offer "evidence" of their good work, while they provided us with the raw material for ours. In spite of these "hopes," I had a growing sense that there was a larger set of responsibilities still unmet, ones that suggest that these traditional notions of researcher/community reciprocities were not sufficient, if we were to consider ourselves to be feminist researchers. A question that arose was whether my/our unease could be attributed to this particular context in which the stakes are so high and the issues are both personal and urgent. I began to feel the pull of participant stories, including the personal risks that participants took in sharing their views and experiences with such candour. In turn, I wanted my/our "response" to their stories to reflect this urgency.

These wonderings gave rise to a desire to interrogate the nature of our responsibilities and the possibility of/for reciprocity within the structural and social constraints engendered by and through academic research frameworks. A later encounter with Fraser's (1995, 2001) and Feldman's (2002) work encouraged Tara Gibb and myself (now both doctoral students) to reconsider our earlier notions of responsibility and reciprocity from another perspective, and so to our first two Rs we add two more, redistribution and recognition.

Negotiating Four "R's": Responsibility, Reciprocity, Redistribution, and Recognition

That research is a fraught process is neither a novel nor a surprising observation; therefore, one would expect that a research field crowded with interests, positionalities, and competing political and social agendas would necessitate multiple negotiations. Crowding this particular research field were varying and sometimes conflicting responsibilities and concerns about reciprocity, both of which were complicated by issues of status inequity (Fraser 1995, 2001). As mentioned in the preceding section, we (graduate researchers) were torn by our sense of responsibility to our mentors, to the larger state-funded project, and to our community partners. While our mentors carved out a learning and working space in which there was a great deal of reciprocity – that is, there was an equitable distribution of give and take – we graduate researchers struggled within the confines of the project to create a similar space within the immigrant service organizations. The limitations imposed by the research question and the funding guidelines thwarted our attempts to fulfill our felt responsibility to engender reciprocity in our relationships with the managers and administrators of the ISOs with whom we worked. Gradually, methodological and ethical issues emerged that we later related to issues of recognition and redistribution and the challenge of taking these up within traditional research frameworks.

We wanted to recognize the important work of the organizations, and ensure that this work was accurately represented and acknowledged by government representatives who were overseeing this project, in order to instigate policy changes that would directly improve the conditions of immigrant women. However, we were acutely aware of the power imbalances in the research process, which we understood to be the product (at least partially) of government policies relating to the provision and foci of settlement resources, including resources for educational programs. We began to realize that issues of inequitable resource allocation dictated by funding protocols were accompanied by a lack of recognition of the skills and knowledge of immigrant women. This misrecognition, we have since concluded, requires at the very least a critique of liberal multiculturalism that privileges notions of the good (implicit in the Canadian multicultural ethos) over an ethos of justice (which calls for a redistribution of both economic goods as well as the transformation of structures and systems that privilege some identities over others). In this section, we explore how researcher responsibility and reciprocity might be reconsidered within Fraser's (1995, 2001) and Feldman's (2002) call for what we have come to think of as a redistribution of recognition.

Canadian multicultural policies have their focus on supporting the integration of immigrants and cultural others into the social and economic fabric of Canadian society (Government of Canada 1985; Etherington 1994). Within this ideological context it is understood that the good is constituted through an affirmational model with a focus on policies and practices that embody fairness and that "seek to eliminate unjustified disparities between the life-chances of social actors" (Fraser 2001, 23). Fraser (1995, 2001) and Feldman (2002) have critiqued earlier articulations of recognition-based models of justice (including affirmational models) that underpin, for example, Canadian multicultural polices. Their counter-proposal calls for a "break with the standard 'identity' model of recognition," which requires "group-specific cultural identity" (Fraser 2001, 23). According to Fraser, models such as the Canadian multicultural example reflect an affirmational approach to identity and justice issues, leaving underlying and oppressive structures intact. Fraser calls for attention to and redress of "institutionalized patterns of cultural value [that] constitute some actors as inferior, excluded, wholly other or simply invisible, hence as less full partners in social interactions" (2001, 24). She proposes a critical theory of recognition that contains the possibility for highlighting the shortcomings of liberal multicultural policies. This, we argue, provides an important framework to untangle the complex relationships that were, at the very least, an irritant to funders but that at their worst perpetuate a system that privileges the statist voices at the expense of, in this particular case, our community partners, both administrators and immigrant women.

Acutely aware of the power imbalances present in this myriad of research relationships, one way the researchers sought to address issues of inequitable resource allocations was to discuss the implications of funding protocols for our relationships with our community partners. As holders of research funds and working on behalf of potential program funders (HRDC), we became acutely, and at times, uncomfortably aware of the potential for our research to become complicit in perpetuating ongoing structural and systemic inequities. Our community partners were also well aware of the inequities in resource allocation within formal scholarly research contexts. Through persistent, if indirect messages, the administrators of the immigrant service organizations we were working with made clear their understanding that our research funding could be partly directed to their organizations as one way of redressing these inequities. For example, one administrator requested monetary compensation for the clients of her agency who agreed to participate in interviews in order to remunerate clients' time and transportation costs. The research team agreed that this compensation should be extended to all the research sites, and grocery vouchers were purchased according to the limits established through funding protocols. On another occasion, one administrator requested a significant sum of money to be gifted to the agency to compensate for their staff's time and efforts to accommodate our research presence within their organization. This caused a significant dilemma for the research team because such a request could not be extended to the other agencies involved in the research.

What began to rankle was the insufficiency of our efforts to minimize inequity and a desire to reconceptualize the ethics of research conducted with vulnerable community partners. Recalling our sense of the research relationships as fraught, we turn to the work of Fraser (1995, 2001) and Feldman (2002), which offers a way to rethink and relink issues of racism (including gendered racism) and distributive justice in the case of researching immigrant service organizations and essential skills. This rethinking of our research relationships and their implications for inequity is oriented towards bringing to the surface how notions of citizenship and belonging are embedded in particular funding and research frameworks and the implications of these understandings on "the struggle for recognition" in which immigrant women are involved (Fraser 1995, 68).

Responsibility within the Context of a Redistribution of Recognition

One persistent question in our many discussions throughout this project (and, indeed, long after its conclusion) relates to multicultural policies and their impact on funding for research into issues of immigrant retraining and integration. Did the research question presume the need for "wholesale transformation of societal patterns of representations, interpretation and communication that would change everybody's sense of self," or did it perpetuate acceptance of unequal social relations (Fraser 2005, 73)? Either way, neither state multicultural nor funding policies are neutral sites, but rather, they embed and are imbued with particular notions of what constitutes either the just or the good as they relate to economic and cultural well-being.

Historically, economic and cultural well-being, or redistribution and recognition, have been theoretically separate and, according to Fraser (1995), falsely dichotomized. Fraser proposes reclaiming recognition such that it becomes an integral part of justice for the purpose of addressing inequities perpetuated by the subordination of particular identities. While a full discussion of her argument is beyond the scope of this chapter, what we wish to make use of here is Fraser's expanded notion of injustice to include "cultural or symbolic injustice ... rooted in social patterns of representation, interpretation and communication" (71). In the past, economic goods have been the focus of distributive theories of justice, and Fraser's work has been to expand understandings of distributive justice to include recognition as a social good that also requires equitable distribution. We understand Fraser's project to be about the redistribution of recognition – and that recognition in this framework relates to overcoming the subordination of particular identities and racial or cultural groups. The purpose of linking recognition with distributive justice is to achieve "reciprocal recognition and status equality," which constitutes a shift from liberal understandings of recognition to a critical orientation (Fraser 2001, 24).

Fraser (1995, 2001) has diagnosed multiculturalism's malaise as being the result of its focus on *the good* rather that *the just*. That is, in multicultural policies the corrective is not to be found in transforming institutions and thereby social relations (the just), but in calling for the liberal subject to freely choose what has been described as morally correct (the good), which may require corrective measures such as education and training. But, as Fraser points out, without the transformation of structures (which includes funding and human resource policies) dominant discourses about what is moral or good are continuously reinscribed within complex discursive fields. In spite of multicultural policy, in spite of programs to expand the Canadian imaginary to include those racialized as Other, the founding imaginary (that of two European nations with only a recent and cursory nod towards the original people of Canada) appears to be reflected in the original research question, *"How can the voluntary sector be an effective instrument for delivering programmes for the acquisition of essential skills to Canada's immigrant populations?"* The question presumes that so-called essential skills are both essential to, and found lacking within immigrant populations. What has been misrecognized is the possibility that immigrant (women) may already possess these skills sufficiently to gain professional employment and that they may already possess other equally essential skills for employment. In the absence of such recognition, immigrant women are denied distributive justice (access to good employment, jobs commensurate with their skills, and so forth) and are reduced to deficient individuals requiring remediation in order to fit within the Canadian national imaginary.

Recognition and redistribution are often constructed as a binary in activist and academic circles. Fraser (2001), however, argues that this binary is a false antithesis: "Justice today requires *both* redistribution *and* recognition; neither alone is sufficient" (2001, 22, original emphasis). How do researchers recognize the voices of our community partners and ensure that research resources are distributed equitably, particularly when research questions are predetermined by funding agencies imbricated with and in a liberal multicultural framework? Fraser's notion of parity of participation opens possibilities for considering different avenues for transforming research protocols in policy contexts. Fraser (2001) explains that current models of identity recognition, those following the ideas of Charles Taylor (1994) and Axel Honneth (1992, 1995), construct bounded single group identities with little consideration for the multiplicity of people's identities and the social institutions and social relations that contribute to identity construction. Fraser proposes, instead, the status model, which suggests that recognition comes not from group-specific identity but from "the status of group members as full partners in social interaction" (24). By recognizing status rather than identity, researchers can examine the effects of institutionalized patterns of cultural value that impede parity of participation in the research process.

Relinking the Political and the Social

In our efforts to resituate our research work as political work, we appreciate
the tools that Fraser (1995, 2001) and Feldman (2002) have provided us,
which enable the possibility of linking identity, class, and race within a
critical framework and reconsidering the possibility of research (even that
which is funded through problematic statist frameworks) as an overtly political act. Feldman (2002), building upon Fraser's (1995, 2001) work, emphasizes that civil society is an important site of and for political struggle.
Researchers, community-based service providers, and clients of these services all have a potential role to play in critiquing and challenging policies that
perpetuate an unequal distribution of recognition. Political/recognitional
injustice may be institutionalized through government policies, but the policies are also enacted in civil society.

According to Feldman (2002), the role of civil society in perpetuating both
misrecognition and distributive injustice cannot be left un-interrogated.
Funding policies and research associated with civil society are both an instrument and a reflection of state ideologies and, consequently, become the
site of struggles for justice. As stated earlier, federal multicultural policies
reflect a liberal ideology that presumes an Enlightenment subject, a division
between the public and the private, and presumes the state as having a role
in protecting individual liberty while ensuring an economically competitive
marketplace (Feldman 2002; Foote 2003; Olssen 2003; Young 2001). We
view federal policies, such as the HRDC polices relating to essential skills
funding and training, as affirming this view of the individual, the state, and
their relationship to each other.

Early on in the project, together with our community partners, we recognized that the Essential Skills policies were flawed because they failed to
interrogate these basic assumptions, and they failed to consider that the
deficit did not rest within the individual immigrant, but with our (Canadian)
understanding of what counts as knowledge, skills, and credentials. Based
on our reading of the data with Fraser's (1995, 2001) and Feldman's (2002)
work in mind, we suggest that both the flawed essential skills policy and the
funding programs that emanated from it reflect a distributive injustice that
misrecognizes immigrant women in problematic ways that result in what
Feldman (2002) refers to as political exclusion.

As feminist researchers who situate our work within critical frameworks,
we are drawn to use language and analyses that engage with issues of justice,
not morality. In the case of this particular research project, the essential skills

question is more about retrofitting immigrants with the skills deemed necessary by the dominant culture than about interrogating institutionalized subordination (Fraser 2001). Issues of racism and other forms of discrimination are not factored into this research question; the barrier between immigrants and good jobs resides within each individual immigrant and her or his possession or lack of one or more of the nine essential skills identified by HRDC.

There is abundant theory and scholarly work relating to the production of immigrants, and immigrant women, as a subordinate class (Bannerji 2000; Ng 1996; Razack 2004; Thobani 2000). As Thobani has observed, "the social construction of immigrant women as outsiders is also simultaneously a parallel process constructing Canadians as insiders in relation to, and in opposition to this Other" (2000, 282). Thus, as we have noted in our research, even women who were not working-class in their countries of origin (i.e., who had the benefit of one or more university degrees and were working in professions in their countries of origin) were not immune from being the excluded. In this regard, Fraser's framework for addressing the inequitable distribution of recognition is helpful. Immigrant women's identities, misrecognized, underrecognized, and denied status, do not require remediation through reskilling or retraining; rather, what is required is that the state attend to policies and practices that deny both distributive and recognitional justice. Fraser has clearly stated that both race and gender have often been problematically relegated to identity politics, which sidesteps issues of status and reciprocity. In retrospect, we conclude that our unease with the research frame dictated by the funders was due to our lack of capacity to either adequately challenge the funding structure and liberal framework that gave rise to the research question or to voice and enact our own nascent feminist epistemologies. The knowledge communicated to us by the women we worked with in the community could find little space to answer back to the research question. In that space, their call for justice was not heard within the liberal framework. The women we spoke with were talking about justice – of the redistribution of recognition and of economic resources. Our research question, as originally framed, filtered out their voices, leaving a silence that demanded new questions to interrogate the injustices and inequities experienced by immigrant women – while still considering the salience of identity. In this regard Fraser's (1995, 2001) work has provided us with an important epistemic and ontological framework with which to both analyze and formulate research questions in collaboration with community partners.

Concluding Reflections

In reflecting upon our research relationship with the immigrant women's organizations, we have come to realize that the frustration that they (and we ourselves) felt within the confines of the funded research question is that it perpetuated misrecognition, which includes misrecognizing the site of the injustice. It is not the lack of retraining programs that was stinging but rather the lack of recognition that most of the women who are targets for training already possess the essential skills, with the exception of fluent "Canadian English." If we are to engage in collaborative research, as many protocols now state researchers must do, this means significantly altering the parameters of how policy research is conducted. Integration of immigrants and cultural Others means providing status as full partners in social interaction, including the negotiation of research agendas. However, under current multicultural discourses that inform policy research, this is not the case. One possibility is conceiving research from the standpoint of status recognition and redistribution. In state-funded policy research, this would entail all members involved in the research process (community agency administrators, agency clients, academics, policy makers) to be present at the table to negotiate the research questions and the allocation of resources. All constituencies will no doubt have different interests and questions that they want addressed; therefore, the research process will continue to be fraught with struggles and stings. We are not suggesting this is a detriment. Instead, it holds the possibility of all parties being recognized and given the opportunity to communicate. Susan Bickford (1996) explains that the prospect of this is disconcerting because what we hear may require us to reconsider and let go of entrenched assumptions about ourselves and others. It is also scary because it challenges us to think differently about the systems in which we are entangled and complicit. Although it is daunting, taking up Bickford's challenges for those of us who engage in research foregrounds our responsibility to attend to the tangled web of relationships that constitute the research project and to scrutinize the ways in which our research processes mitigate or perpetuate recognitional injustice.

ACKNOWLEDGMENTS

The research on which this chapter is based was supported by funding from the Social Sciences and Humanities Research Council of Canada grant no. 854-2003-10. We wish to acknowledge the academic researchers with whom we conducted the two case studies discussed here: Tara Fenwick and Katie Campbell. This chapter is based on "Tangled Nets and Gentle Nettles: Learning in Immigrant Service Organisations," a paper authored by T. Fenwick, K. Campbell, T. Gibb, E. Hamdon, and Z. Jamal, and published in, *Proceedings of SCUTREA [Standing Conference for University Teaching and Research in the Education of Adults]* (Leeds: The Media Services, University of Leeds, 2006), 105-11.

REFERENCES

Bannerji, Himani. 2000. *The Dark Side of the Nation: Essays on Multiculturalism, Nationalism, and Gender.* Toronto: Canadian Scholars' Press.

Beyene, Dawit, Carrie Butcher, Betty Joe, and Ted Richmond. 1996. "Immigrant Service Agencies: A Fundamental Component of Anti-Racist Social Services." In C.E. James, ed., *Perspectives on Racism and the Human Services Sector: A Case for Change,* 171-82. Toronto: University of Toronto Press.

Bickford, Susan. 1996. *The Dissonance of Democracy: Listening, Conflict and Citizenship.* Ithaca, NY: Cornell University Press.

Etherington, Brian. 1994. *Review of Multiculturalism and Justice Issues: A Framework for Addressing Reform.* Ottawa: Department of Justice.

Feldman, Leonard. 2002. "Redistribution, Recognition, and the State: The Irreducibly Political Dimension of Injustice." *Political Theory* 30(3): 410-40.

Foote, John. 2003. *Federal Cultural Policy in Canada.* Prepared for the Council of Europe/ERICarts "Cultural Policies Compendium." http://www.oas.org/oipc/english/documentos/polpercentC3percentADticasculturalescanada.pdf.

Fraser, Nancy. 1995. "From Redistribution to Recognition? Dilemmas of Justice in a Postsocialist Age." *New Left Review* 212: 68-93.

–. 2001. "Recognition without Ethics?" *Theory, Culture and Society* 18(2): 21-42.

Gannage, Charlene. 1999. "The Health and Safety Concerns of Immigrant Women Workers in the Toronto Sportswear Industry." *International Journal of Health Services* 29(2): 409-29.

Gibb, Tara, and Evelyn Hamdon. 2010. "Moving across Borders: Immigrant Women's Encounters with Globalization, the Knowledge Economy and Lifelong Learning." *International Journal of Lifelong Education* 29(2): 185-200.

Gibb, Tara, Evelyn Hamdon, and Zenobia Jamal. 2008. "Re/Claiming Agency: Learning, Liminality and Immigrant Service Organizations." *Journal of Contemporary Issues in Education* 3(1): 4-16.

Government of Canada. 1985. *Canadian Multiculturalism Act.* RSC 1985, c C-24 (4th Supp).

Guo, Shibao. 2002. "An Interpretive Study of a Voluntary Organization Serving Chinese Immigrants in Vancouver, Canada." Unpublished PhD diss., University of British Columbia, Vancouver, BC.

Henry, Frances, Carol Tator, Winston Mattis, and Tim Rees. 2000. *The Colour of Democracy.* Toronto: Harcourt Brace.

Holder, B. Saddeiqa. 1998. "The Role of Immigrant Serving Organizations in the Canadian Welfare State: A Case Study." Unpublished PhD diss., University of Toronto.

Honneth, Axel. 1992. "Integrity and Disrespect: Principles of a Conception of Morality Based on the Theory of Recognition." *Political Theory* 20(2): 188-89.

–. 1995. *The Struggle for Recognition: The Moral Grammar of Social Conflicts.* Cambridge: Polity Press.

HRDC (Human Resources Development Canada). 2002. *Knowledge Matters: Skills and Learning for Canadians: Canada's Innovation Strategy.* Document SP-482-02-02. Ottawa: Author.

HRSDC (Human Resources and Skills Development Canada). 2004. *Meeting the Challenge: A Guide to Working with Essential Skills.* Government of Canada HIP-007-03-04. Gatineau, QC.

Mojab, Shahrzad. 1999. "De-skilling Immigrant Women. *Canadian Woman Studies* 19(3): 123-28.

Ng, Roxana. 1996. *The Politics of Community Services: Immigrant Women, Class and State.* Halifax: Fernwood Publishing.

Olssen, Mark. 2003. "Structuralism, Post-Structuralism, Neo-Liberalism: Assessing Foucault's Legacy." *Journal of Educational Policy* 18(2): 189-202.

Razack, Sherene. 2004. "Imperilled Muslim Women, Dangerous Muslim Men, and Civilised Europeans: Legal and Social Responses to Forced Marriages." *Feminist Legal Studies* 12: 129-74.

Reitz, Jeffery. 2003. *Occupational Dimensions of Immigrant Credential Assessment: Trends in Professional, Managerial and Other Occupations, 1970-1996.* Toronto: University of Toronto, Munk Centre for International Studies.

Scott, Katherine. 2003. "Funding Matters: The Impact of Canada's New Funding Regime on Nonprofit and Voluntary Organizations – Summary Report." *Canadian Council on Social Development.* http://www.ccsd.ca/pubs/2003/fm/summary-fundingmatters.pdf.

Taylor, Charles. 1994. "The Politics of Recognition." In *Multiculturalism: Examining the Politics of Recognition.* Princeton, NJ: Princeton University Press.

Thobani, Sundera. 2000. "Nationalizing Canadians: Bordering Immigrant Women in the Late Twentieth Century. *Canadian Journal of Women and the Law,* 12(2): 279-312.

Young, Judy. 2001. "No Longer 'Apart'? Multiculturalism Policy and Canadian Literature." *Canadian Ethnic Studies* 33(2): 88-116.

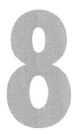

Challenging Policies for Lone Mothers
Reflections on, and Insights from, Longitudinal Qualitative Interviewing

PENNY GURSTEIN, JANE PULKINGHAM, AND SILVIA VILCHES

In this chapter, we reflect on the implications of using a longitudinal qualitative research design to investigate the everyday experience of lone mothers in the context of neo-liberal welfare reform. We also consider the methodological and ethical complexities of this research as a feminist methodology for critical policy analysis. Longitudinal research involves repeated data collection/generation with the same group of research participants over an extended period of time, and as such, it is a relatively resource-intensive and, therefore, less often used research design. Even so, longitudinal quantitative data sets are increasingly available for policy research, whereas longitudinal qualitative research designs remain much less common. As a result, this study provides an opportunity for insight into a topic that is more typically examined through short-term research designs. Using the Income Assistance Project, based in Vancouver, Canada, as a case study, we investigate how our approach situates knowledge and our understanding of the negotiated trajectories of women's lives (Dyck and McLaren 2004; Naples 2003; Fine et al. 2000).[1] We examine, with hindsight, the strengths, limitations, and dilemmas of doing critical policy-relevant research on poverty (Goode and Maskovsky 2001). As Shaw (2004) and Marshall (1999) suggest, a critical feminist policy analysis focuses on the ways in which policies are positioned as gender neutral by ignoring the wider socio-political context within which recipients live. Following in these footsteps, we see ourselves as writing "between poor communities and social policy at a time of

Right-wing triumph," seeking "to be taken seriously by both audiences," and, as a result, struggling with what it means "to think through the power, obligations, and responsibilities of social research" (Fine et al. 2000, 108).

Our research points to the power of longitudinal qualitative research to give voice to impoverished women, allowing for a more nuanced understanding of the disjunction between policy and women's everyday lives, in particular their life-course and socio-political trajectories. But our research also points to the complexities and unintended consequences of applying what Maskovsky (2001) calls policy-driven or policy-relevant criteria in the design of the research. Building on, and extending Thomson and Holland's (2003) analysis of the normative tensions that inhere in longitudinal (qualitative) research pertaining to change, or what may be called progress, we reflect how, over time, the participants in our study benefited from the research, and how extended research time enabled a more complex analytic understanding of the research participants.

Turning a critical eye inward, we also look at what extended time in the data-generation phase (via both multiple and iterative interviews) enabled us to learn from silences, including sample attrition, for policy making. We consider how the longitudinal qualitative methodology presented a unique opportunity to engage in critical reflection on questions of representation and identity, an opportunity that would not have arisen in a cross-sectional or one-shot qualitative interview design. We also reflect on the insights gained from this critical reflection regarding the limitations of the categorically driven policy identification of women with young dependent children as merely women with dependent children of a certain age, revealing the ambiguities in such categorization.

The Research Context

Welfare Reform in British Columbia

Welfare reforms in British Columbia, similar to those implemented elsewhere in Western developed nations (Brodie 2004; Jenson 2004; Kingfisher 2002), are part of a broader set of activation policies designed to move people from welfare to work. In 2002, a new Liberal Party government introduced sweeping changes to British Columbia's welfare system, setting stricter limits on access and reductions in supports. One of the reforms, time limits on welfare entitlement, or the so-called two-in-five year rule, was unprecedented in Canada. This rule, which limited eligibility for welfare to two years in any five-year period for recipients who were classified as "expected to work," marked a significant departure from previous welfare legislation in British Columbia and elsewhere in Canada by invoking welfare time-use – rather than needs-based (e.g., income, financial means, family circumstances, health, disability, employment) eligibility criteria. Implementation of welfare time limits was modelled after welfare reforms implemented in the United States in 1996 (the Personal Responsibility and Work Opportunity Reconciliation Act). In British Columbia, parents with dependent children (the majority of whom are lone mothers) were especially affected by the reforms, because the legislation changed the timing of work expectations for parents with dependants: parents were deemed employable when their youngest child was three years of age, reduced from seven years of age.[2]

The Income Assistance Project: Purpose and Design

The Income Assistance Project, which began in 2003, was designed as a longitudinal study to examine the impact of welfare reforms, in particular, the time limits to welfare benefits, on lone mothers with young children. Our objectives, to provide immediate policy-relevant information, as well as a more general analysis of welfare reforms and their implementation in neo-liberal contexts, played into methodological decisions.[3] While we wanted to understand women's everyday lives from their own perspectives, we were also interested in the interplay of their lives with policy objectives. We wondered how women negotiated the imposition of the time limit rule and what would happen when, or if, they reached the end of the time limit. Thus, we focused on action and counter-action between the women and policy constraints as they negotiated the new range of program expectations and requirements. We were also curious about any potential effects of changes to other support services, which were implemented simultaneously with the income assistance reforms. Thus, while the data came to us through the everyday experiences of the women, we pursued an inquiry into the effects of the neo-liberal agenda of program cuts, balanced budgets, and the so-called activation of BC's citizens.

An underlying tension in the research was between the here-and-now demands of policy-relevant research, which the women desired, and the benefits of more abstract academic critiques, which may have longer-term effects. This tension was heightened by the longitudinal nature of the project, which demanded that interviewers/researchers maintain the relevancy of the research to participants over time, but also, perhaps, that participants sustain themselves as research "subjects." It is this latter dilemma that provides an opening for deconstructing the complexities of feminist longitudinal interviewing, especially as we consider those who did not remain in the study for the duration.[4]

Sampling and Recruitment Implications

The desire to focus on everyday experience and to examine the impact of policy changes meant that a small sample and a longitudinal design were ideal. We designed the sample so that we could see the impact of crossing two welfare policy thresholds: (1) into the expected-to-work (ETW) category, when the youngest child turned three years of age, and (2) over the two-in-five year time limit, which would be reached two years later, when the youngest child turned five years of age. Women recruited at the start of the study self-identified as lone mothers receiving what was classified as temporary assistance. At the time of recruitment, half of the women had a youngest child between eighteen months and three years of age, while the other half had a youngest child between the ages of three and six years. In all, seventeen mothers were scheduled for interviewing six times between May 2003 and January 2007, with individual consent renewed at each interval.[5]

In addition to welfare timelines, we were also interested to know more about urban Aboriginal women's experiences. While the incidence of lone parenthood is rising for the population as a whole, the incidence of lone parenthood is more common among Aboriginal peoples (37.1 percent on-reserve and 40.2 percent off-reserve Aboriginal families) than it is among non-Aboriginal peoples (21.7 percent of non-Aboriginal families) (BC Stats, 2005). In addition, Aboriginal lone parents are more likely to live in extreme poverty, at almost one-half the income level of their non-Aboriginal counterparts. Thus, we aimed to recruit one-half of the sample as Aboriginal; nine of the seventeen mothers in our study self-identified as Aboriginal.

Another important aspect of the design was the geographical focus of the sampling. East Vancouver is an area of both concentrated poverty and service provision. Women in our study faced the double dilemma of an increased need to draw on services provided by a range of voluntary sector organizations who themselves were subject to government funding cutbacks. Given that our goal was to enable women to talk freely about this dual dilemma without feeling that the information they shared in the interviews might jeopardize relationships with agency facilitators, our recruitment strategy deliberately bypassed agency-based access. This latter strategy turned out to be a key factor in establishing relationships in which the women felt free to construct, or author, their own narratives, as shall be discussed below.

The interview guide was open-ended, and like Naples's (2003, 147) US research on lone mothers receiving Aid to Families with Dependent Children (AFDC), it was designed to elicit mothers' narratives about their everyday lives and "the demands placed on them by policy implementation criteria." The interview guide we used started with one main open-ended question: "I am really interested in learning from you about your experience of living on Income Assistance. Maybe we can start by you telling me about the daily routine of one day in your life in the last week? The day you choose to describe can be a typical or usual one, or it could be an atypical or unusual day." Subsequent interviews were designed to enable the mothers to expand on what was going on in their lives in the months between interviews, and to allow the interviewers to follow up on particular issues/themes that emerged in prior interviews.

A Focus on Time

Multiple Sequential Interviewing

The study was focused on the tensions with the specific social timetable dictated by the new welfare policy, especially the requirements to seek employment, hinged as it was to the aging of the child. Thus, time, including participant time, policy time, and interviewer time, as well as social timelines, became organizing analytic and experiential frameworks. Since our study paralleled the implementation of the welfare reforms, our research occurred in current time, that is, our research participants, and we as researchers, were consumers and participants in a grand social experiment.

The study was initiated in 2003 to catch the occasion, in 2004, on which the province's first wave of welfare recipients would reach the two-in-five year time limit. This threshold was passed at about the time of the third interview for those participants in our study whose youngest child was three years of age or older at the time of recruitment. The other half of the participants in our study, whose youngest child was under three at the start, also reached their first transition threshold at the time of the third interview, moving from the category of "temporary assistance, excused from work search obligations" to the "expected to work" category. The time leading up to this threshold was fraught with anxiety for the participants, but also for the interviewers, who were concerned for the women who were already struggling on reduced resources.

The interviewing format was not just longitudinal, but also iterative, organized in a multiple-sequential fashion (Pulkingham and Kershaw 2008). The term *multiple-sequential interviewing,* used by Ortiz (2001), captures two important dimensions of the interviews that we conducted: (1) the opportunity to conduct numerous or repeated interviews and (2) repeat interviews that have a time/order or longitudinally oriented purpose. The repetition permitted us an understanding of the interactions over time of the impact of policy changes in the context of mothers' lives. From an analytic point of view, this highlighted the tensions between the relative fit (and more often the gap) between the mothers' lives and the policy prescriptions. The difference in the shifting nature of the gaps across the group provided the opportunity to examine the premises of particular normative expectations about life-course trajectories, including specific transitions such as education, work, and family formation, given the different mothers' experiences and identities. This cross-sectional, or comparative aspect, was enriched by the multiple interview format, which permitted depth of analytic understanding to build on the women's own aspirations and achievements within the constraints and supports of their individually constructed lives.

One of the advantages and complexities of multiple interviewing is that it permits (though does not guarantee) the development of rapport over time. Among other things, this enables the researcher and research participant to pace when and how personal information is shared (Oakley 1981; Kezar 2003), alleviating some of the discomfort that participants and researchers may feel. In addition, in the context of being welfare recipients, participants in this study were well acquainted with the process of having to tell and retell their story or circumstances to bureaucratic gatekeepers and overburdened support workers (Robertson and Culhane 2005); this was an issue to which the researchers were highly sensitized. As Pulkingham, Fuller, and Kershaw (2010) suggest, the research interviews were distinguished from the bureaucratic encounters, because the women were taken seriously as authors of their own lives (Kiesinger 1998; Ortiz 2001). It was for this reason that it became particularly important that we had not recruited women through any particular service agency. As Dyck and McLaren observe, how and what stories are listened to matters: Following in their footsteps, the interviews we conducted were also intended to create both "conditions under which women [were] able to construct accounts of their concerns and experiences as 'facts' that need to be heard, both in terms of being important to listen to for policy-makers" (2004, 514-15) and to add to research about the difficulties experienced by impoverished lone mothers, in particular, Aboriginal mothers. The process of listening became an exercise in which our views of participants' contexts gradually reshaped over time, and this process informed the development of different kinds of analytic categories that challenged policy concepts and assumptions embedded in public discourses.

The multiple, iterative nature of the longitudinal interview design constituted its own challenging micro-politics, which gave rise to our later reflections in this chapter on why some women withdrew from the study. The intention was to provide an opportunity for the research participants to tell and retell their stories over time in such a way as to afford the researcher "a much deeper understanding of the seasonal cycles" (Ortiz 2001, 197) and the complexity of participants' lives, experiences, accounts, and explanations (Millar 2007). However, this design also put a tremendous responsibility on the researcher, and the participant, to maintain boundaries or manage tensions in the face of expectations, such as life-course transitions, that might build over time. As Cohen (1997) notes, what is being reflected to the interviewer is both a construction of, and a resistance to, what the participant believes public discourse about people *like them* is about, and maintaining a coherent identity over time may cause confusion over their identity (identity fatigue) or dissonance for the participants.

The multiple-sequential interviews also heightened the opportunities for critical self-reflection on what we observed, experienced, and attended to through our own lens. These recurring opportunities for checking our assumptions challenged the research team's multiple disciplinary gazes. This interacted with another kind of timeline tension, between participants' perceptions of power vested in the research team to effect change, our community partners' investments for the purposes of advocacy, and the academic requirements for conceptual rigour. Some participants, like "Andrea," recognized the opportunity that "hopefully something positive comes out of it" for lone mothers.[6] "Jeanie" also expressed her motivation to use the research as an instrument of advocacy, but further, as an unofficial community spokesperson, she saw the interviews as an opportunity to effect change on behalf of her friends and community:

> I actually know a few people right now who would probably like the same thing, you know, to open up. Like, there's a few of us that have this problem with welfare. Like, I've said this to you before, right? If a single mum goes

out and works, we get dollar for dollar taken, but then you get people who are on disability, and they get the extra four hundred dollars a month, and they're allowed to make five hundred dollars a month and they don't get dinged for it. (Jeanie, Round 6)

Jeanie, thus, expressed the complexity of her representation and participation amid the contexts she was juggling, engaging herself and the researchers in societal power differentials.

Thomson and Holland (2003), as well as Fine et al. (2000, 215), document these tensions, which speak to the instrumental desires of research:

Many of the women and men we interviewed both recognized and delightfully exploited the power inequalities in the interview process. They recognized that we could take their stories, their concerns, and their worries to audiences, policy makers, and the public in ways that they themselves could not, because they would not be listened to. They (and we) knew that we traded on class and race privilege to get a counter-narrative out. And so they "consented." They were both informed and informing.

Jeanie's interest in changing policies that impact her life is indicative of tensions that we experienced by asking people to participate in policy-focused research that might not result in material policy change in the short term. This tension is not unique to research: it occurs in many policy processes that involve public participation, including advisory boards, community associations, and the work of policy think tanks. As McNutt and Marchildon reflect, "to have direct influence suggests one actor is capable of convincing another actor to follow a suggested course of action. However, considering the nature of democracy and the numerous players involved in trying to influence government policy action, crediting an institution or actor as responsible for any one particular outcome is unreasonable. Unlike the government ministries, all of which exercise power, the policy analysis industry is engaged in policy dialogue" (2009, 220). But in a research context where we set out to comment on policy, our limited ability to deliver concrete policy solutions does raise questions about the implications of asking participants to comment on their lives over time. This particular dilemma adds additional complexity to the goals of feminist critical policy analysis, in that not only is policy critique held central, but so, too, is empowering women by translating their concerns in an effective and timely manner.

The expectation to create "timely" policy-relevant research also came from the community partners. These community-based research organizations tend to conduct and disseminate research in a much more expeditious manner than the academic partners who must negotiate within the time-tables and requirements of academic funding agencies, research ethics boards, and refereed journals. Tensions were created with the community partners when it became evident that there were lengthy negotiations required within the research team to arrive at common understandings, and with the ethics approval process at the various academic institutions involved (particularly pertaining to protection of confidentiality while providing financial compensation for those who participated in the research), that lengthened the time it took to get the research underway. These tensions were partially resolved with the production and media release of a report of the study's significant findings.[7]

Strengths and Limitations of Multiple Interviewing within a Longitudinal Qualitative Design

One of the ways in which we have evaluated our research strategy was to reflect on what participants told us about their experiences of being interviewed, through unprompted or unsolicited feedback, and in the last interview, by providing participants the opportunity to reflect on what they felt were the benefits of the research and the interviews. As Thomson and Holland (2003) note, there are several ways in which participants may benefit and use the research situation.

The women who remained in the study thought that it had been interesting, and valuable, to have an opportunity to "check in" with someone twice a year to reflect on their own lives, but we realize that these reflections still occurred within the context of the interviewer-interviewee relationship and, therefore, were subject to the constraints that participants may have felt in the interview situation. Potential and likely constraints included the perceived power differential, the growing sense of relationship and connection, and possibly, the modest compensation and expenses reimbursement, which were significant to their household income. However, for "Olivia," for example, having someone to talk to about her life was an enormous support and helped with her loneliness and isolation:

> Like I said, I feel good when I talk to you. I really do. And I feel comfortable.
> I feel relaxed. But when I was sick, you know, I'd go home bored, and start

thinking, and I would cry, right? Because nobody else listened to me, and [I have] nobody else to talk to. And I'd start thinking about my son or my childhood or my parents. Mom, why aren't you here? Stuff like that, right? (Olivia, Round 6)

Olivia did not feel as free to talk about her problems in other settings:

I don't trust anybody, to be honest. Like I said, when they talk, it goes this way, back that way, back this way, and comes back [to me]. (Olivia, Round 6)

This emotionally supportive feeling was also expressed by "Natalie," who talked about how she valued the interviews and how they motivated her:

I really like it because I'm sitting down here at table, and you're willing to hear my problem. And you pay me to listen [to that]! You pay me, so when I go home I get motivation from what I say. And my story's behind [closed doors] and nobody will know. [And when] I go and cook for my kid, I say, "Well, I like people to hear what I say." I like the interviews – they should be continued. Because since I talk to you I get a little bit encouraged and I [move on]. And then I say, "Oh, in six months [she] is going to come and we're going to talk," and I have things to say that I want you to see [that are different]. But when I met you, I was down; whining, complaining. But right now I'm strong. Maybe next [time] I [will] have a job, things. Maybe in ten years from [now] I will win the lottery! (Natalie, Round 6)

Natalie's reflection on why she enjoys the interviews, quoted above, identifies the complicated dynamic of interviews organized around policy dilemmas. The instrumental desire to help others, or to effect change, is articulated here in her desire to be able to report progress, not only for herself, or to meet welfare requirements, but also to please the interviewer. Although Natalie completed all six interviews and expressed regret when they were ending, Natalie also clearly wrestled with the apparent gulf between the material and social circumstances of her life as set against normative expectations and her own aspirations. Given insight through her struggles, it is instructive to reflect on the possible reasons why mothers did drop out over time in the study.

Thomson and Holland (2003) reflect on the challenges of policy change as a potential disincentive to longitudinal qualitative interviews, speculating that because there is a normative element in the continuity of longitudinal interviews, those who do not have progress in normative terms may feel disinclined to continue. Thomson and Holland wonder whether this dynamic might have contributed to sample attrition in their study. Similar concerns arise in our research. While our motivation and intention was to locate women's lives and agency at the centre of the analysis, for some of the mothers it appears that an unintended consequence of tracking policy effects may have been to reinforce rather than counteract the weight of normative expectations, the same issue that was reflected by Natalie, but perhaps with negative consequences for those who were unable to meet perceived expectations. This led us to reflect on the issue of attrition.

At midpoint, one and a half years in, sixteen participants had completed three interviews. By the end, though, five of seventeen participants were no longer participating. Attrition is to be expected in any longitudinal study, especially with a sample that is potentially more difficult to reach or to stay in touch with (more mobile, without reliable telephone access, etc.). But often the issue of attrition (particularly in quantitative studies) is treated as simply a sampling problem, impinging on the inferences that can be drawn from the study, but not given analytic attention. In our study, for some participants, a sense of stalled progress and the lack of anything to report between interviews are clearly evident. For example, in the third interview in which "Marissa" participated, she expressed feeling progressively more blue about the fact that she had nothing to report between interviews. At the time of the fourth interview, she indicated to her interviewer that she did not need the support of government or other programs anymore. For Marissa, God was her salvation, and she expressed this in a concrete way: God was going to find a job for her. Clearly, for Marissa, not only did the interviews seem to underscore a sense of personal failure, but ultimately, the policy-focused interviews ceased to be relevant at all.

We would speculate that for the other participants who dropped out, the question of relevance, and more specifically, resonance, also surfaced, but in a different way. As described above, the sample was predicated on the policy-driven age-based social timetabling of mothers' lives, organized around the age of the youngest child. Built into this timetable is the assumption that the reason for the interrupted employment, and reliance on welfare, is the birth and/or presence of a young child. This builds in an assumption that (lone) motherhood is the central organizing feature that brings these women to welfare. Even though our intention was to query this presumed centrality, the sampling strategy relied on policy-driven categories. These norms were evident in the descriptions provided at the time of the first interview, as well as through the screening questions asked during re-cruitment. Yet, for four of the women who dropped out of the study,[8] re-course to welfare had nothing to do with the birth of their children. At the beginning of the study, these four women identified that their youngest was between the ages of three and six years, and three of the four self-identified as Aboriginal women.[9] For these participants, who had been in receipt of welfare for a relatively long time (ranging from eight to sixteen years; on average, for twelve years), we may speculate that the focus on the intersec-tion of policy and mothering ultimately failed to capture the complexities of their relationship to the welfare system and their core identities.

Fine et al. address a parallel concern with the analytic ramifications of what might appear, at first sight, to be "just" a sampling issue. In their re-search, the sampling problem appeared in the form of not being able to recruit comparable numbers of "'equally poor' and 'equally working-class'" racialized groups (African American, Latino/Latina, and so-called white) (2000, 112). But as Fine et al. conclude, what may appear to be a sampling issue (comparable numbers of different categories of participants) or a sup-posed sampling problem (in our case, sample attrition) "is revealed as con-stitutive of the very fabric of society," providing important analytic insight (113). For our part, in addressing the issue of for whom the research was designed and for whom we were engaging in the research, as Fine et al. put it, we have to conclude that our research possibly failed to fully resonate for some of the women for whom mothering represented only a fraction of their relationship to welfare or of their identity, or for whom the concept or experience of mothering did not meet normative expectations.

As an example, first of the relevance and nature of mothering as an iden-tity, and then of the conflict with material circumstances, one of the Aboriginal women who withdrew, "Anne," started the study with a confusing statement about the number of her children, declaring her youngest to be between three and six years of age. As the interviews evolved, she gradually revealed that she had a youngest child who was under three, some children in permanent foster care, some placed with a relative, and some that she was trying to co-parent in a shared custody arrangement. Thus, although Anne was a mother several times over, and actively cared for her children by sup-plying resources as she could, visiting and worrying about them, her income assistance status was changed to "single, expected to work" about halfway through the study. Once her welfare status changed, the chances of her being able to regain custody diminished, because she was not eligible for a shelter amount that would enable more than rooming-house accommodation.

Over the course of the study, Anne therefore became, once again, an ostensibly childless adult. Although the interview questions were open-ended, Anne was fully aware that the focus of the study was on how mothers coped with the welfare-to-work expectations. Thus, the repeated interviews were reminders of the absence of her children from her life, as well as a normative challenge to her identity as a mother. Like some of the other women who withdrew, a seemingly unconnected event precipitated loss of contact with the interviewer; but the event itself was indicative of the life of a woman for whom mothering was not the central problematic. We can see that the welfare policy bifurcated Anne's identity temporally into mother and then not-mother, categories that we inadvertently replicated in the interviewing context.

The complex relationship of motherhood to welfare experiences, and the complicated relevance of the focus on motherhood for some participants, also raises a different, although parallel (and relevant) point, one that Newman (2001) makes regarding the importance of fully contextualizing the issue of welfare reform for those about whom, and for whom, research is conducted. As Newman argues in relation to the long-term effects of welfare reform in the United States, welfare reforms, even drastic ones, do not necessarily represent a unique event in the lives of the poor; rather, their reality is an existing and highly complex survival strategy in which new welfare reforms are simply the latest in a litany of bureaucratic rules and rule changes that govern their lives, disentitling them or making welfare access more difficult. The welfare reforms themselves may be less salient than other aspects of having to rely on or turn to welfare for support, and experiences of living in poverty, more generally. This insight applies to the situation of the mothers we interviewed, and it is amplified for the women who self-identify as Aboriginal.

When applied to the Aboriginal women's lives, the timelines of the welfare-to-work policies must also be set against the colonial timelines that are still in play for Aboriginal people today. What is evident in our study is that policy history and family history affected these women individually and form part of the historical timeline that helps make the urban/reserve divide (cf. Lawrence 2004). For example, three of the Aboriginal-identified women were raised in foster families. All three indicated a pattern of familial disenfranchisement and legal disentitlement through child protection removal, which was experienced by many Aboriginal peoples in the mid-twentieth century (Fournier and Crey 1997; Shewell 2004). As Collins (1998) points out, race and gender are never separate categories. The family histories of the Aboriginal women were imbricated with past colonial policies that had severed these women's mothers from their reserve communities when they married non-registered Aboriginal men or non-Aboriginal men. At the same time, some of the Aboriginal women talked about extreme violence on the part of their parents; one woman talked about battling the demons when her mother "came out of her" and she struck her own children, against her better judgment and desires ("Nancy," Round 2). For her, as for others whose mothers had lost their children, the complications of colonial policies, poverty, and gender combined to create a living legacy that was still being played out in their own and their children's lives.

The analysis of Aboriginal women's stories or narratives challenged us to listen to and follow their lead, highlighting the gendered as well as racialized nature of poverty for all the women. For example, as we looked at the impact of regulations that instructed Income Assistance staff to tell women to go to friends or family for support before coming for an emergency grant (Gurstein and Vilches 2009), we observed that this failed to acknowledge the depth of poverty in the whole Aboriginal community, as well as the disenfranchisement that women, in particular, had experienced. As Tait (2001) has pointed out, the construction of fragility and risk interacts with gender blindness in policy to make Aboriginal women even more vulnerable to ongoing intervention.

This differential impact of welfare restrictions and colonial policies on the Aboriginal community, and Aboriginal women in particular, lifts our attention from the impact of supposedly neutral welfare policies on individual women to the categorical impact at the societal level on women as a class. This effect at the societal level was most potently expressed in respect to urban Aboriginal women during a focus group that was hosted at the Aboriginal Mother Centre in East Vancouver, where an agency administrator said:

> And that's where we are in 2007, and it's gotten worse since October of 2006 [because] many more of our kids have been apprehended at huge rates. Yet the government is saying the statistics are down. That's for the non-Aboriginal side. In Vancouver Coastal [health] region in 2002, we had 43 percent of our Aboriginal children in care. To October 2006, which is the latest statistics we've been able to get, 75 percent of Aboriginal children were in care. And you ask yourself why, and we're going through this as our services here at the Mother Centre are reduced, the services to the Moms,

and the amount of support they receive has been reduced. (Participant, Focus Group 2)

Seen from this perspective, welfare reform is yet another injury in a long history of state policy injuries that continue to affect Aboriginal peoples. Considering the proportion of lone mothers who are Aboriginal, and the complex reasons for their deep poverty, these comments alert us to the potentially damaging effects of supposedly gender-blind policies. Methodologically, researchers are called on to push the boundaries of received understanding, especially in a potentially exploitative context of difference and intersectionality (Anderson et al. 2003; Haig-Brown 2003). The longitudinal iterative format, in particular, gave us time to hear and understand the depth of historical time, which was still active for the Aboriginal women, in spite of the wide array of individual differences between them. Thus, although some women had access to resources that others did not have access to, as a group, these women struggled within the context of different dimensions of gendered aspects of colonial history, whether that was poverty that drove women into the sex trade, historically or today, or literacy issues arising out of differentiated schooling experiences, or federal policies that continue to provide a barrier to enfranchisement.

Discussion and Conclusion

In setting out to do research that provides a feminist critical policy analysis of welfare reform in British Columbia, we challenged the historical and policy conditions that create differential impacts for women. In challenging the constructed silence generated by assertions of equality and gender-neutrality within policy, we highlighted the way discourses around motherhood and children interact with race and gender to create highly distinct patterns of impact for lone mothers. We deliberately tried to avoid the style of policy-relevant research, especially some evaluation research, that runs the risk of leaving unexamined the merits of the policy goals themselves, thereby undermining the ability of the research to "contribute meaningfully to the reversal of current patterns of economic polarization and social inequality" (Maskovsky 2001, 472).

At one level, when examined through the lens of feminist critical policy analysis, our research does help uncover the way in which policies are far from gender neutral in the manner in which they are designed to move lone mothers into the workforce, how they use state apparatuses to exert control over women's sexual and reproductive lives, and how they constrain women's autonomy in other arenas as well (e.g., education and employment opportunities, community engagement, and familial support). For the researchers, our study offered an opportunity for the critical depth of understanding needed to make compelling, nuanced statements on policies that affect lone mothers' lives. For the participants, it provided a needed space for reflection on their experiences. As Bensimon and Marshall (2003, 347) note, "feminist theory and language of critique" can provide a firm basis "to command forceful critique of continuing cultural exclusions." The use of multiple interviews within a longitudinal qualitative research design was a powerful tool for pushing the boundaries of knowledge creation by focusing data generation on the trajectory of women's lived experiences in their own voices.

At the same time, the tensions in this research are equally compelling. Demonstrated by the attrition of participants from the study, the relevance of the research was not necessarily sustained for all of the women; over the long term, some clearly did not identify with the embedded assumptions. By initially aligning the focus of our research with a particular piece of policy legislation, a particular set of welfare reforms, and a particular group of recipients, we inadvertently played into "policy relevant" categorizing, which Maskovsky (2001) alerts us to, in this case, lone mother/not lone mother, welfare recipient/not welfare recipient, and new/not new welfare rule. These categories inadvertently served to decontextualize the lives of many of the women for whom we had initiated the research. In addition, we were also challenged to translate and disseminate findings in a timely manner to affect social policy. One component of our approach was to make the research findings accessible through our collaboration with community partners who have linkages to the non-academic community sector and public organizations, yet these partnerships also heightened analytic tensions with what constituted "a timely manner." Nevertheless, we did publish with our community partner, as well as meet with policy bureaucrats. But together, we (academic researchers and community partners alike) struggled with the narrowed policy scope of what it means to be relevant in the world of policy makers, including both politicians and bureaucrats, and what relevance means without compromising our responsibility to the women we interviewed.

The constraints of the research design raise issues about who the real audience is and how to engage decision makers in the experiences of women. But, in spite of the limitations of our research, we found that the longitudinal qualitative research design played an important role in manifesting what is often overlooked and disregarded, because even with the best of intentions to do things differently, we had to wrestle with the insidious ways in which the policy focus threatened to limit the scope of the research. The objective of conducting feminist critical policy analysis helped us make sense of the bureaucratic structures and the webs of personal and community entanglement that confine women to poverty and marginalization and committed us to representing the perspective of women's strategies and struggles in negotiating their social and physical environments.

NOTES

1 The Income Assistance Project is a longitudinal qualitative study of the impact of welfare reforms, and cutbacks to other social services and supports, implemented in British Columbia beginning in 2002, on lone mothers with young children. The study was funded through the Consortium for Health, Intervention, Learning, and Development (CHILD), a SSHRC MCRI project.
2 During the two-year transition phase, once their youngest child had reached three years of age, parents who were expected to work also faced much more onerous work search requirements, to be pursued through an "employment plan" drawn up with the ministry responsible for welfare (then called the Ministry of Employment and Income Assistance).
3 The research was undertaken by a multidisciplinary team of academic researchers partnered with researchers from two community-based policy think tanks – the Social Planning and Research Council of British Columbia and the Canadian Centre for Policy Alternatives, BC Office.
4 Five participants did not remain in the study for the duration: one participant declined to be interviewed after the first interview, while the remaining four participants could not be contacted, either because their contact information was no longer valid or because they did not respond to telephone messages, after the fourth interview.
5 In total, we conducted eighty-eight interviews.
6 All names are pseudonyms to protect the identity of the study's participants.
7 See Gurstein et al. (2008).
8 All four of these participants had dropped out by the fourth interview; one had dropped out after the first interview.
9 Altogether, eight of the women interviewed in our study had turned to welfare before they had had any children of their own. They did so for a variety of reasons, including fleeing violence, ill health, looking after (fostering) younger siblings, unemployment, and longer-term receipt of welfare. Of these women, four did not participate in our study for the duration. None of these four women explicitly told us that they did not want to continue in the research; rather, they could not be reached at the time of the fifth and sixth interviews, either because the contact information we had for them was no longer valid (which speaks to the instability of their living situation and the fact that they could not or chose not to update us as to their

whereabouts) and/or because they did not return our telephone calls. While four women who also had been in receipt of welfare before they had children did remain in the study for the duration, one notable difference between the women who "stayed" and those who did not is that among the former each one had a child who was under three years of age at the time of the first interview and/or went on to have another child during the course of the study. All of these women were mothering very young children.

REFERENCES

Anderson, Joan, JoAnn Perry, Connie Blue, Annette Browne, Angela Henderson, Kousbambbi Basu Khan, Sheryl Reimer-Kirkham, Judith Lynam, Pat Semeniuk, and Vicki Smye. 2003. "'Rewriting' Cultural Safety within the Postcolonial and Postnational Feminist Project." *Advances in Nursing Science* 26(3): 196-214.

BCStats. 2005. *British Columbia Statistical Profile of Aboriginal Peoples, 2001: With Emphasis on Labour Market and Post Secondary Education Issues* [Electronic Version]. Victoria, BC: BC Stats, Ministry of Management Services. http://www.bcstats.gov.bc.ca/data/cen01/abor/tot_abo.pdf.

Bensimon, Estela M., and Catherine Marshall. 2003. "Like It or Not: Feminist Critical Policy Analysis Matters." *Journal of Higher Education* 74(3): 337-49.

Brodie, Janine. 2004. "The Great Undoing: State Formation, Gender Politics, and Social Policy in Canada." In Barbara A. Crow and Lise Gotell, eds., *Open Boundaries: A Canadian Women Studies Reader,* 2nd ed., 87-96. Scarborough, ON: Prentice-Hall.

Cohen, Jodi R. 1997. "Poverty: Talk, Identity and Action." *Qualitative Inquiry* 3(1): 71-92.

Collins, Patricia Hill. 1998. "Intersections of Race, Class, Gender, and Nation: Some Implications for Black Family Studies." *Journal of Comparative Family Studies* 29(1): 27-36.

Dyck, Isabel, and Arlene T. McLaren. 2004. "Telling It Like It Is? Constructing Accounts of Settlement with Immigrant and Refugee Women in Canada." *Gender, Place and Culture* 11(4): 513-35.

Fine, Michelle, Lois Weis, Susan Weseen, and Loonmum Wong. 2000. "For Whom? Qualitative Research, Representations and Social Responsibilities." In Norman K. Denzin and Yvonna S. Lincoln, eds., *Handbook of Qualitative Research,* 2nd ed., 107-31. Thousand Oaks, London, and New Delhi: Sage Publications.

Fournier, Suzanne, and Ernie Crey. 1997. *Stolen from Our Embrace: The Abduction of First Nations Children and the Restoration of Aboriginal Communities.* Vancouver: Douglas and McIntyre.

Goode, Judith, and Jeff Maskovsky. 2001. Introduction. In Judith Goode and Jeff Maskovsky, eds., *New Poverty Studies: The Ethnography of Power, Politics and Impoverished People in the United States,* 1-34. New York: New York University Press.

Gurstein, Penny, Michael Goldberg, Sylvia Fuller, Paul Kershaw, Jane Pulkingham, and Silvia Vilches. 2008. *Precarious and Vulnerable: Lone Mothers on Income*

Assistance. Burnaby BC: SPARC, 23 pp. (Dec.). http://www.sparc.bc.ca/resources-and publications/category/44/income-assistance?start=20.

Gurstein, Penny, and Silvia Vilches. 2009. "Re-Visioning the Environment of Support for Lone Mothers in Extreme Poverty." In Marjorie Cohen and Jane Pulkingham, eds., *Public Policy for Women: The State, Income Security, and Labour*, 226-47. Toronto: University of Toronto Press.

Haig-Brown, Celia. 2003. "Creating Spaces: Testimonio, Impossible Knowledge and Academe." *Qualitative Studies in Education* 16(3): 415-33.

Jenson, Jane. 2004. *Canada's New Social Risks: Directions for a New Social Architecture*. Ottawa: Canadian Policy Research Networks.

Kezar, Adrianna. 2003. "Transformational Elite Interviews: Principles and Problems." *Qualitative Inquiry* 9(3): 395-415.

Kiesinger, Catherine. E. 1998. "From Interview to Story: Writing Abbie's Life." *Qualitative Inquiry* 4(1): 71-95.

Kingfisher, Catherine, ed. 2002. *Western Welfare in Decline: Globalization and Women's Poverty*. Philadelphia: University of Pennsylvania Press.

Lawrence, Bonita. 2004. *"Real" Indians and Others: Mixed-Blood Urban Native Peoples and Indigenous Nationhood*. Lincoln: University of Nebraska Press.

Marshall, Catherine. 1999. "Researching the Margins: Feminist Critical Policy Analysis." *Educational Policy* 13(1): 59-76.

Maskovsky, Jeff. 2001. "Afterword: Beyond the Privatist Consensus." In Judith Goode and Jeff Maskovsky, eds., *New Poverty Studies: The Ethnography of Power, Politics and Impoverished People in the United States*, 470-82. New York: New York University Press.

McNutt, Kathleen, and Gregory Marchildon. 2009. "Think Tanks and the Web: Measuring Visibility and Influence." *Canadian Public Policy* 35(2): 219-36.

Millar, Jane. 2007. "The Dynamics of Poverty and Employment: The Contribution of Qualitative Longitudinal Research to Understanding Transitions, Adaptations and Trajectories." *Social Policy and Society* 6(4): 533-44.

Naples, Nancy. 2003. *Feminism and Method: Ethnography, Discourse Analysis, and Activist Research*. London: Routledge.

Newman, Katherine S. 2001. "Hard Times on 125th Street: Harlem's Poor Confront Welfare Reform." *American Anthropologist* 103(3): 762-78.

Oakley, Ann. 1981. "Interviewing Women: A Contradiction in Terms." In Helen Roberts, ed., *Doing Feminist Research*, 30-61. London: Routledge and Kegan Paul.

Ortiz, Steven M. 2001. "How Interviewing Became Therapy for Wives of Professional Athletes: Learning from a Serendipitous Experience." *Qualitative Inquiry* 7(2): 192-220.

Pulkingham, Jane, Sylvia Fuller, and Paul Kershaw. 2010. "Lone Motherhood, Welfare Reform and Active Citizen Subjectivity." *Critical Social Policy* 30(2): 267-91.

Pulkingham, Jane, and Paul Kershaw. 2008. "The Income Assistance Project: The Intersections of Welfare and Life Course Transitions among Lone Mothers." Paper presented at Lone Mothers and Welfare to Work Policies: Insights from

Longitudinal Qualitative Research, International Symposium, Simon Fraser University (at Harbour Centre), Vancouver, 26-28 Sept. 2008.

Robertson, Leslie A., and Dara Culhane, eds. 2005. *In Plain Sight: Reflections on Life in Downtown Eastside Vancouver*. Vancouver: Talonbooks.

Shaw, Kathleen M. 2004. "Using Feminist Critical Policy Analysis in the Realm of Higher Education Policy: The Case of Welfare Reform as Gendered Educational Policy." *Journal of Higher Education* 75(1): 56-79.

Shewell, Hugh. 2004. *"Enough to Keep Them Alive": Indian Welfare in Canada, 1873-1965*. Toronto: University of Toronto Press.

Tait, Caroline L. 2001. *Aboriginal Identity and the Construction of Fetal Alcohol Syndrome*. Report No. 10. Montreal: Division of Social and Transcultural Psychiatry, Department of Psychiatry, McGill University.

Thomson, Rachel, and Janet Holland. 2003. "Hindsight, Foresight and Insight: The Challenges of Longitudinal Qualitative Research." *International Journal of Social Research Methodology* 6(3): 233-44.

White Cow*boy*, Black Feminism, Indian Stories

PAUL KERSHAW

Prologue

Small Small Cowboy Paul. That's what the community researchers called me.

The "Cowboy" part is easy to explain. I live on Homecoming Farm, where I raise horses and grow food in a Vancouver suburb that most now refer to as Pitt Meadows, British Columbia, Canada. But in the absence of any formal treaty, it remains Katzie Territory – something cowboys have historically ignored.

The "Small Small" part of the name arose from idle chit-chat. All but one in the conversation belonged to minority ethnocultural groups in Canada, and many explained that their names have "meaning" in other languages. Several expressed surprise that I had no idea what my name meant. Suitably embarrassed, I consulted a "baby name" book. Paul, it turns out, means "small"; and William, my middle name, can be interpreted as "little."

Being called "small" once isn't great for the white *male* ego. Emphasizing with repetition any lack of size risks psychological scarring. Did my parents not read the available name books?

When I later shared the etymology of my name with the others, Dong Dong, a colleague of Chinese ethnic descent with an apparent knack for poetry, announced (and giggled) that I would henceforth be referred to as Small Small Cowboy Paul.

I do regularly wear a cowboy hat and boots on the farm. But for academic purposes, I prefer to emphasize the *boy* in *Cowboy*. It's subversive. White adult males rarely refer to themselves as "boys." Since the term infantilizes its subjects, many white men (and women) refer(red) instead to males of colour as "boys" to communicate their white racial power. In response, I have for some time illuminated this white privilege by juxtaposing my "whiteness" with my "boyness." Doing so unnerves other "white men," and draws explicit attention to the intersection of my race and sex no matter who is the audience. I have subsequently embraced the "Small Small" moniker because it accentuates this effect. And when theorizing about the legacy of colonialism in Canada, emphasizing the small *boy* in *Cowboy* is helpful for disrupting dominant cowboy and Indian stereotypes.

The "boy" name also appeals to me personally. Too many *men* are violent, especially towards women; and too many men neglect a wide range of important social responsibilities, including caregiving, in order to free-ride off the hard work of diverse groups of women. Do I really want to develop into that? I'm not convinced. Nor is my partner. So she refers to me as her "boy"; not her "man." I take it as a compliment and strive to develop qualities that others may not regard as "manly."

That's the story behind my name.

But Did You Ever Hear the One about a White Cowboy Doing Black Feminist Research Inspired by Indian Stories?

That's the important story in this chapter. It's not one you often hear. And some may even question whether a white, affluent male can do black feminist methodology, or engage ethically in research with Aboriginal peoples. But I think the answer to such questions is, and ought to be, yes. You may agree after you hear this white boy's story about the organization of the Care, Identity, and Inclusion (CII) Project.

In this story, the white cow*boy* works in collaboration with women of colour and Aboriginal women through community-based research to place their expertise at the centre of theory building. It's a story that demonstrates why and how this was done, and it explores some of the methodological and ethical tensions involved in order to share insight about how to commence collaborations, allocate funding to moderate power dynamics and promote community priorities, and use community expertise to develop analytic frameworks, as well as integrate women who do not speak the majority language.

The story resists the inclination to revel in the self-flagellation of confessing ethical duplicity or exploitation, which some imply is inherent to feminist community-based research. In so doing, this small cow*boy* follows

Kamala Visweswaran (1994, 40) in conceding that such research entails a necessary loss of innocence among feminist academics. We cannot escape the power differentials that exist between the researcher and researched, the scholar and the community member, particularly when the feminist academic is a white, affluent male. But Visweswaran is careful to emphasize a loss of innocence – that is, far greater sensitivity to *the risk* of betraying feminist principles, along with fear of feeling betrayed by those principles – rather than insist on the *impossibility* of conducting feminist community-based scholarship. This distinction is critical and motivates the CII story to focus more pragmatically on methodological decisions that scholars can make to, at the very least, minimize the ethical tensions.

The CII Project starts with a well-documented fact about Canada, and many societies: caregiving is undervalued. Our governments do not count the social reproduction to which caregiving contributes in GDP or other standard measures of economic progress. Canada is recognized by UNICEF (2008) as an international laggard in terms of family policy. Those who shoulder primary responsibility for caregiving are generally un(der)paid, and risk economic, social, and political marginalization. Men, while a heterogeneous group, do disproportionately little care work, reaping economic and political privileges from this unencumbered status. As a consequence, many men also enjoy proportionately less fulfillment from caregiving.

In response, this white cow*boy* is keen to illuminate what is socially valuable about caregiving, and to identify the policy implications of this value, in part, to remedy the gender division of labour. His involvement in the CII Project contributes to this objective.

The Muse

Patricia Hill Collins is the CII Project's muse. In her seminal book *Black Feminist Thought: Knowledge, Consciousness, and the Politics of Empowerment* (1991) and her subsequent essay "Shifting the Center: Race, Class and Feminist Theorizing about Motherhood" (1994), she reveals the analytic and ethical imperative to shift the experiences of women of colour to the centre of theory building. One reason this shift is necessary is because we only learn about key political dimensions of caregiving when we listen to those who provide care, while they cannot count on the public sphere to validate their group identities. When schools, the media, and other public institutions ignore or misrepresent the identities of racialized ethnic groups, caregivers in those groups must compensate. They must guard their children against ubiquitous messages that brand their children as less valuable, with less potential. As Collins explains, minority ethnic caregivers confront the responsibility to cultivate "a meaningful racial identity in children within a society that denigrates people of color" (1994, 57). By instilling within children the confidence to trust their own self-definitions, parents equip their offspring with "a powerful tool for resisting oppression" (Collins 1991, 51).

Caregiving? A tool for resisting oppression? This and more, Collins suggests: The struggle to instill a proud ethnocultural awareness within their children reveals that some women's "subjective experience of ... motherhood is inextricably linked to the sociocultural concern of racial ethnic communities – one does not exist without the other," Collins argues (1994, 43). The implication is that some domestic care functions as resistance to oppression that stretches well beyond the particular homes in which the work is performed, because it contributes to a broader project of community development. Minority ethnic mothers contribute to sustaining the self-definition of collective identities, and the collective political agency to which such self-definition gives rise, by working to ensure that their children cultivate a proud affiliation with their cultural history.

This is an enormously important insight about caregiving. If processes of identity formation in domestic spaces foster the ability of some individuals and the social groups in which they are members to claim and exercise power in modern states, then we have new reason to query whether some domestic care should be considered civic and political engagement, and to hypothesize that some "private" caregiving time may be necessary for "social" inclusion (Kershaw 2005, Chapter 6).

There remains, however, little empirical data with which to test the hypothesis. Appropriately privileging experiential expertise, Collins (1994) refers to literature and poetry authored by African American women and other minority mothers to inform her arguments. Other important contributions include that of Dua (1999) and Roberts (1995), who integrate sociohistorical and legislative evidence in their analyses. But, given the relative dearth of data, Small Small Cow*boy* Paul initiated the CII Project to explore further the "private time for social inclusion" hypothesis.

Other People's Questions

Starting with a hypothesis generated from black feminist literatures is critical for any white boy who aims to conduct research in this tradition, or to practise the "reflexivity" recommended by Wolf (1996) and others when selecting projects. Given that my social location is defined in part by my white, affluent, heterosexual, male, and Christian background, I can only conduct feminist research by subverting the norms, values, and questions that are typically privileged in this location in favour of the norms, values, and questions that are prioritized by those who are not so systemically empowered. I exercise this subversion by learning from the likes of Collins and others who recommend alternative questions to ask and answer.

But while an ethical commitment to hypothesis testing may avoid one methodological pitfall, it invites another. A white boy who aims to place the expertise of women of colour at the centre of theory building will not act alone. Yet, collaborative methodologies imply mutual interest in the study topic; interest that reflects community priorities as much as academic pursuits. This poses a serious dilemma. Just how does one generate a project that reflects community priorities when one feels ethically bound to practise reflexivity by investigating a less privileged social group's academic hypothesis?

They Asked First

The route out of this dilemma demands that one pursue collaborations very purposefully. For instance, I set out to find a particular kind of community program, one that promotes caregiver-child time and that was adopted enthusiastically in minority ethnocultural communities. Program participation would thus signal interest in the CII hypothesis; interest that originated from local desires, and thus predated my particular motivation to approach community members with a proposal to collaborate.

In searching for such a program, I was guided by a disturbing recognition: Aboriginal people in Canada may be uniquely aware of the political significance of caregiving for identity because colonizers specifically deployed caregiving as a strategy for assimilation and the destruction of Aboriginal cultures. The "traditional" academic understanding of the Indian Residential School System, as labelled by Trevithick (1998), implies that Canadian governments benignly intended the schools to assimilate Aboriginal children in their best interest. The revisionist understanding maintains that the schools were central to an aggressive strategy to eliminate Aboriginal cultures in Canada. Regardless of which view you favour, both make clear that governments organized caregiving to function as a colonial mechanism. Indeed, the forcible disruption of familial and community patterns of caregiving in favour of state-sanctioned residential schools proved such a potent colonial intervention that many speak of the schools as a system of cultural genocide (e.g., Chrisjohn and Young 2006).

Out of respect for this unique expertise about caregiving, I sought a community partner that would embrace the indigenous epistemology to which Thomas King refers in *The Truth about Stories: A Native Narrative*. According to King (2003, 2), "The truth about stories is that's all we are." His observation is enormously important when planning data collection. For if, ontologically, all we are is stories, then we ought to prioritize collecting data through narrative approaches.

But the epistemology to which King refers is not just important methodologically. His truth about stories gets at what is important about "private time for social inclusion." We *are* the stories we tell ourselves, or that others tell us. We self-define with stories, and thus stories are integral to the agency to which our self-definitions give rise. This, too, is Collins's point. That is why she recognizes that parents of colour must guard their children from messages that risk implying they are less worthy. Such caregiving will include storytelling to resist the racism that they or their loved ones encounter.

Guided by these selection criteria, I identified the programs HIPPY and Aboriginal HIPPY, or Home Instruction for Parents of Preschool Youngsters. Both organize around the principle that facilitating the caregiver-child bond within the family home is a powerful intervention for increasing parental agency and child success. And both use stories, often told in children's books, to focus the parent-child time.

While HIPPY internationally targets lower-income families in general, the program in Canada has proven popular with recent immigrants and Aboriginal communities. Among the latter, Aboriginal organizers queried the value of integrating a program that evolved from a non-Aboriginal context. After careful deliberation, organizers modified the curriculum to feature stories germane in their First Nations as part of a strategy to enhance caregiver-child time to contribute towards cultural revitalization; and they renamed the program so that *Aboriginal* precedes *HIPPY*. The home visitors who work on behalf of Aboriginal HIPPY are members of First Nations, typically from the local community. By contrast, all HIPPY home visitors are immigrant women of colour, who generally share an ethnocultural and linguistic heritage with program parents, and facilitate their participation in a language other than English. Home visitors in both programs work part-time. They meet weekly during the school year with participant families to support parents to nurture relationships with their children, preparing them for the school system in Canada; and in the case of Aboriginal HIPPY, with attention to the legacy of Indian residential schools. Given these program characteristics, HIPPY and Aboriginal HIPPY represented ideal potential partners with which to explore the value of a research project that would be citizen-led and foster local capacity, while testing the "private time for social inclusion" hypothesis urged by literature associated with Collins.

As luck would have it, the HIPPY Canada director, Debbie Bell, is a superb adult educator committed to social justice who, when the CII Project was still an idea rather than reality, also was on the Faculty of Continuing Studies at Simon Fraser University (SFU) in Vancouver. Tammy Harkey, the Aboriginal HIPPY director, was employed in the same SFU unit and a powerful Musqueam voice for justice in Aboriginal communities. Since our paths crossed occasionally at other local research meetings, I did not have to start from square one in terms of relationship building. This is no small matter, since relationships are key to collaboration.

My first conversations about CII were with Debbie, as we shared a cab from an airport to a hotel where we'd be attending the same academic conference. Because Debbie is a white, affluent woman, I broached the idea of collaboration during the cab ride only informally, asking to discuss directly with the HIPPY home visitor staff their interest in collaboration. Debbie facilitated the latter meeting by inviting me to a staff lunch among home visitors.

Time Is Money

The lunch was an hour long. No funding was available to convene a longer event and pay HIPPY staff for their valuable time. One hour is clearly not sufficient to initiate genuinely trusting relations *and* solicit feedback from ten different people about their interest in co-leading a research project. It did prove long enough, however, for the HIPPY home visitors to confirm two things: first, that their program is organized around the idea that supporting parent-child time is a potent social justice intervention for minority community members; and second, that the HIPPY team members were interested in research that may show that their program contributes to social justice in ways that they do not typically emphasize. As a result of the lunch, the HIPPY staff sanctioned my pursuing research funds with which we could carry on the conversation about collaboration in more detail.

Where would the funds come from? Traditional academic granting agencies like the Social Sciences and Humanities Research Council (SSHRC) of Canada make only modest collaborative planning grants available. But modest funds would not be sufficient to convene and pay ten staff and two directors for their time to evaluate what, if any, research idea to pursue, and how to pursue it. Free-riding on HIPPY paid time was also not an option, because the two programs already struggle to sustain funding.

Debbie found the solution. She forwarded to me a call for proposals from the Government of Canada Social Development Partnerships Program (SDPP). The competition solicited applications specifically "for funding to sustain and strengthen the capacity of the national, social non-profit sector through organizations that address the social development needs of ... children and their families ... includ[ing] social inclusion and/or early learning and child care" (http://www.hrsdc.gc.ca/eng/community_partnerships/sdpp/index.shtml).

This unique call for applications meant that we could submit an application for funding to support HIPPY and Aboriginal HIPPY in delivering their services *because* the programs would provide the site for innovative research. Debbie, Tammy, and I negotiated that we would collectively prepare a funding application in which we would capitalize on my academic credentials as principal investigator (PI) to justify the need for the research, while as co-investigators they would take the lead to develop a project budget, co-develop the work schedule, and identify deliverables. This division of labour was both purposeful and, I would argue, respectful: respectful because I already get paid to write and submit research grants; they don't. Assuming those who are not paid as researchers should collaborate equally in writing research grants on their own time disregards programmatic pressures.

We went for broke, requesting $900,000 over three years to support existing HIPPY programs in Vancouver and three Coast Salish First Nations, while also injecting funds to initiate new HIPPY programs in Toronto and Montreal. This funding would subsidize the salaries of Debbie and Tammy; partially pay Aboriginal HIPPY and HIPPY home visitor wages, in recognition that their programmatic time would become the setting for CII research, while also paying for additional employment for home visitors. The additional paid time would free them to be trained, and they could then serve as community researchers who would engage the expertise of the parents already participating in their programs. By comparison, modest time/teaching release funds were allocated for the small white cow*boy* in his PI role.

In its wisdom, SDPP responded by awarding our proposal $740,000 over the three years. Short a $160,000, Debbie adjusted our proposal by eliminating Montreal as a research site.

Put Your Money Where Your Mouth Is

Now that we were adequately funded, authentic collaboration could begin. It started with the decision that all funds would be allocated directly to HIPPY and Aboriginal HIPPY to manage, in keeping with their directors' preferences. In contrast to the colonizing practices implicit in so much scholarship, the decision to empower the programs with fiduciary responsibility aimed to mitigate the power differentials that typically favour university partners when collaborating with communities, and to ensure that the research progressed with due concern for the priorities of community members.

This was no easy decision. One year into a tenure-track position, the SDPP grant was the first earned by Small Small *Cowboy* Paul as a principal investigator. And it was three-quarters of a million dollars! Now, nearly five years along that track, it remains by far the largest grant I have received as a PI, since standard research competitions from SSHRC typically pay only $100,000 or so over three years. The decision was made more complicated still because the HIPPY and Aboriginal HIPPY programs were formally located at Simon Fraser University. This meant SFU would claim credit for the funding when measuring its success in external grant competitions, and it would also deduct a 10 percent administration fee for the privilege. From the standpoint of my university, the University of British Columbia (UBC), these optics and payments were far from ideal, as my associate dean made clear after learning about the funding arrangement.

The funding arrangement was also not ideal for me. When evaluating its professors for promotion, UBC only counts funding that its researchers bring through UBC financial services. None of the CII funding figured formally in my tenure and promotion review beyond what departmental colleagues elected to emphasize. This is the case despite the fact that the funding contract with the Government of Canada made explicit that I was the principal investigator on the project.

While not ideal for me personally, the allocation of fiduciary responsibility to HIPPY and Aboriginal HIPPY has been advantageous for the community partners. This funding arrangement without doubt gave financial security to the programs for the duration of the CII project. As HIPPY Canada Board Chair Richard Stursberg wrote in a letter to me:

> Your understanding the centrality of the community-based partner was unprecedented with your original decision, as principal investigator, to leave the research contract with the community partner – HIPPY Canada. Your

willingness to stick with the decision when HIPPY Canada moved from SFU will provide HIPPY Canada a desirable stature as a stand alone non-profit and enable us to build our credibility with federal government agencies over the long run.

Just as important, responsibility for CII research funds empowered the program directors to adapt our research plans in accordance with their priorities: programmatic, research, and ethical. Adaptation was the name of the game from the outset. Tammy, in her wisdom, acknowledged that our funding application had not done enough to position HIPPY home visitors as formal leaders in the project. The risk, she indicated, was that she was the token "executive" Indian and the token "executive" person of colour.

In response, we reworked the funding to invite six home visitors to serve alongside Debbie, Tammy, and me on an executive committee to guide how the team conceptualized care, identity, and inclusion, and to co-organize data collection among minority ethnocultural groups; I do not list the other executives' names because of confidentiality assurances to which I committed in the consent letters they signed. But in so doing, I fail to *name* their contributions, which merits scrutiny by academic research boards (see Reid et al., who explore this issue in chapter 11). The new executive members represented Aboriginal, African, Vietnamese, Latin American, and Chinese ethnocultural backgrounds. As the CII Project evolved, we recognized that our team and sample underrepresented Muslim residents. We later adapted the initial executive committee to add three Islamic community researchers to help organize the project from perspectives attuned to Muslim experiences post-9/11.

Organizing around Their Stories

Empowered by this diverse, talented leadership group, the initial year of the project featured a journal process through which the seven minority ethnocultural members of the executive (all but Debbie and me) and three additional home visitors explored their understanding of the terms *care*, *identity*, and *inclusion*, as well as the interconnections among these concepts. This journalling by the ten women was not planned in the initial grant application. However, the executive decided to devote the first months of the project to journal writing and review out of concern that the "private time for social inclusion" hypothesis would provoke conversations that were riskier for parent participants than the white cow*boy* had initially suggested to funders. The risk, some of my colleagues insisted, is that care is a form a resistance *to discrimination*. No matter how empowering that resistance may be, we are still inviting participants to contemplate when they are targets for subordination. Secure in my white, male, affluent privilege, the women implied that I had not appreciated the potential hurt one suffers when revisiting such experiences; and I certainly wasn't being strategic in thinking people would be attracted to devote time to the project, even if paid, if their experiences of discrimination would be the initial focus.

We therefore adapted the plan, again. The ten minority ethnocultural women who would conduct future interviews for the study elected to explore personally the "private time for social inclusion" hypothesis before approaching other parents. They would do so by writing journals about project themes in contexts where they felt safe. All journalling time was paid for on par with their HIPPY hourly wages. Guided by the recommendations of Aboriginal executive members, the group chose to journal initially in response to the question: Do you or your children have to compromise part of your identity to feel included? Why or why not? Every two weeks for a three-month period thereafter, the ten writers would e-mail journal entries to Small Small Cow*boy* Paul, who would respond with individually tailored questions that invited further exploration of themes raised in each writer's previous submission, while also including common questions for all journal participants. Common questions included: How important is it that your children know your culture or language? How do you create and support identity with your children? And what are the challenges to passing down your culture or language? Journalling thus emerged as an iterative, semi-structured interview that occurred in writing electronically between me and each of the ten home visitors. It simultaneously trained home visitors in the use of computers, e-mail, and word processing, which they would use as interviewers with parents in the next stages of the project.

The significance of this journal process for subverting the risk that my ideas would dominate the project design should not go unnoticed. Guided by King's indigenous story-based epistemology, along with the experienced-based epistemology that is fundamental to many intersectional methodologies (Simien 2007, 265), I used the ten women's journal entries – their stories – to adapt my interpretation of Collins's conceptual framework about caregiving. I then used the adaptation to familiarize home visitors with the associations between caregiving, identity, and inclusion to which their own narratives alluded. Their journal entries thus contributed core content around which community collaborators revised my initial representations of the "private time for social inclusion" hypothesis. The same journal data were used to immerse the Aboriginal HIPPY and HIPPY staff in what *we*, and not just *me*, meant by caregiving, identity, and inclusion. This immersion was critical for the ten women to perform later as data collectors and analyzers, not just serve as expert providers of data. In particular, sharing findings from journal entries enabled greater inter-interviewer consistency as the women took on the role of facilitating semi-structured, qualitative face-to-face interviews with a purposive sample of another seventy parents.

In order to immerse the ten Aboriginal/HIPPY employees, now community researchers, in the project content to which their own ideas were contributing, we relied heavily on the adult education expertise of Debbie and Tammy. I would not engage in another collaboration with community partners in the absence of people who are trained specifically as adult educators: people who know how to use activity, art, video, games, and so on, to teach. These strategies empowered the other executive team members to provide data and leadership about the content of our project in ways they would not have, if we had only relied on academic-style meeting structures and written memos for communication.

Their Interviews

After a year of exploring together the meaning of care, identity, and inclusion, and developing preliminary research questions to ask other participants, the CII Project was ready to move to the next research phase. Parent interviews started in month thirteen of the study, and generally occurred twice every six weeks during a single school year. About thirty-five parents were interviewed in year two; and another thirty-five were interviewed in year three. The ten journal writers recruited all of the participants and conducted all of the interviews.

This research design capitalized on the trust that HIPPY and Aboriginal HIPPY home visitors already enjoy with HIPPY parents. While the trust would allow the interviewers to eventually probe sensitive issues that include experiences of exclusion, our first year of journalling motivated team members to start their interviews by focusing more generically on cultural continuity. To this end, up to thirty-minute conversations about care, identity, and inclusion were added to the end of two out of every six weekly Aboriginal/HIPPY home visits that unfolded in parents' homes. The initial interview in the series began with the question: Is it important to pass on your cultural identity to your children? Why or why not? Subsequent interviews included questions that responded specifically to observations shared by individual interviewees, but also posed common questions for all participants. These included: What, if anything, would be lost if your child does not learn your culture(s)? Where or with whom do you feel like you belong in Canada? Do you encounter discrimination based on your race or ethnicity? And how do you develop a sense of pride for yourself or your children? In the third year, we also invited interviewees to reflect on observations shared by participants in previous interviews in order to perform a qualitative-validity check of our narrative data.

It is worth noting that we only interviewed mothers. This methodological decision reflects the current gender division of labour, which positions women to be more familiar than men with the diverse aspects of social reproduction to which caregiving contributes. But by illuminating further linkages between caregiving and citizenship, our study produced additional evidence with which to question why social policy fails to oblige men to share equally with women the citizenship work inherent in caregiving.

The majority of the interviews with mothers were conducted in their first language, although not the languages of the Aboriginal participants' First Nations. (Aboriginal participants explained that the residential school system had robbed them of the opportunity to learn these languages from their parents and grandparents.) Among participants for whom English was a second language, the six-week routine during the school year went as follows: the home visitor interviewed the parent in the first week; transcribed the interview into the parent's first language in the second week; revisited the parent in a third week to verify the transcript and invite revisions; transcribed the second meeting in week four; and, finally, translated both the first and second meetings into English. The final English transcript was sent to the small cow*boy* to read in order to recommend additional questions for the home visitor to integrate into interviews in the next six weeks of data gathering.

Home visitor fluency in languages other than English was integral to the study design in order to access the experiential expertise of a group of Canadian residents who are less often heard in research about citizenship, identity, and exclusion. Eleven English-Language-Learning parents, however, participated in interviews in English with home visitors. In such cases, the data-gathering process unfolded as described above, with the exception that transcripts produced in week two and reviewed in week three were in English.

A Cow*boy* Guide

Some readers may question just how much the CII collaboration moved the experiences of women of colour and Aboriginal women to the centre of theory building, if the white boy was constantly guiding the questions that such women asked and answered? This is a fair question. Reflexivity is one thing; setting aside entirely one's identity-related predilections and power is another. Still, it is worth remembering that I recommended questions and analyzed all interviews in the light of the home visitors' own journals, along with the feminist framework for theorizing about motherhood proposed by Collins (1994) and by King's (2003) *The Truth about Stories*. Guided by such literatures, I am confident that the role I played in generating interview questions was a strength of the CII study for at least two reasons. The first is methodologically straight forward: by reading all transcripts every six weeks and proposing the next questions, the cow*boy* enhanced inter-interviewer consistency. Given that most of the community researchers were working for the first time as interviewers, some excelled more than others. It was, therefore, necessary to run a quality control over the research process to ensure not only that all interviewers pursued the same themes in their CII sessions with parents, but also that they did so in a way that was sufficiently searching.

A second strength of this methodological design is that it respects (what this white cow*boy* considers) an appropriate division of labour in community-university collaborations. Treating community and academic partners as equals does not entail that they must perform all of the same roles, just as any good feminist will reject a simplistic "equality as sameness" paradigm. The ten Aboriginal/HIPPY employees who became community researchers were content experts, given their lived experience. They also had relations of trusts with participants without which the research could not have been conducted. But their year-long introduction into research design and content analysis during the first phase of our collaboration did not negate my more formal training, nor my knowledge of a broader academic literature. The latter matters when deciding what questions to ask next during interviews, so that data contribute effectively to academic and community debates. Accordingly, the interviewers and I struck a deal. They could ask whatever questions they wanted during the interview, and they could decide not to ask questions that I proposed.

The latter rarely happened. Did interviewer compliance with my suggestions signal ongoing power dynamics? No doubt it did, because I was the only white male on the team, and the only "academic" researcher. Whether these power dynamics also discouraged the ten women from raising additional questions is less clear, although I hope this is not the case. Notwithstanding these limitations, I have no doubt that many CII interviews would have been less probative had I not been guiding them in the light of the interviewers' own journals entries, among other literatures.

Group Analysis – Apart

The small white cow*boy* did not analyze the interviews alone. Home visitors were paid to journal for several hours a week during the summer about their previous year of data collection. In each case, they responded to two questions: What, if anything, did you find surprising in your interviews? And how, if at all, has your thinking about care, identity, and inclusion changed since you started the project? I then used their answers to guide my work with the data. When they found ideas surprising, or changed their thinking because of an interviewee's comments, I took those to be particularly important passages to analyze. When their thinking didn't change, I went back to their journals from the first year of the project to remind myself about what themes they initially emphasized.

This journal approach to community participation in data analysis was not the original plan. We held periodic research meetings at which I intended to present preliminary thematic breakdowns of the data for interviewers to consider. In our first attempt, I showed that narratives shared by many recent immigrants differed substantially from those shared by Aboriginal people. I illustrated this by drawing on journal submissions that the ten interviewers had submitted, in the hope that I would make the point clearer if my colleagues saw the themes articulated in their own words. Their data showed that immigrant participants often referred to Canada in relatively favourable terms as a multicultural country; one where they could, in principle, preserve some parts of their identities while also enjoying more freedom and/or economic security than they did in the countries from which they had emigrated. Aboriginal participants, by contrast, consistently referred to Canada as a place of injustice.

As soon as I made this distinction, however, the group dynamics deteriorated. By using their own words to distinguish points of view, my community colleagues felt I was dividing the room, drawing uncomfortable divisions among our team. They didn't want to continue. "The more we get together, the happier we'll be." That was the implied mantra for group analysis. Accordingly, I pursued the alternative journal strategy for community researchers to share their analyses. But this alternative seriously undermined my hope and expectation that the group would share together, at the same time, in analyzing data. It also reinforced my privilege as the white affluent boy (albeit guided by other epistemologies and the interviewers' own stories) to arbitrate what did and did not count as appropriate interpretations. Had the ten community researchers been in the room with me at the same time, group dynamics would have likely dampened this privilege.

Regrettably, the group divisions anticipated by community researchers once proved prophetic – not because analytic distinctions paved the way for group animosity, but because human beings hold biases even when pursuing social justice together. An Aboriginal colleague had just finished telling that police regularly obstructed the only access to her reserve by performing car inspections and breathalyzer tests. These were police lines that her children had to cross when coming home from a friend's or when their friends' parents were dropping them off. The Aboriginal colleague intended her story to make clear that her community continues to be targeted by authorities who hold negative stereotypes about Indians. But another colleague, an immigrant (it doesn't matter from which region), reinforced these stereotypes by responding in her imperfect English with something like: "I understand why the police target Aboriginals."

The statement didn't come out right. I don't think it is what the second colleague meant. I'm sure it is not what she would have said in one of the two other languages that she speaks fluently. But it was out there; and it was a slap in the face for our Aboriginal team members. They had shared so much in the group by that point, almost two years into the project. Like everyone else in the room, they had allowed themselves to become vulnerable. They trusted that their identities, their group membership, would not be denigrated by team members. That trust was violated.

It took a long time to refurbish group dynamics, and they were never the same. To this day I worry that I let my Aboriginal colleagues down at that moment, once again asking them to contribute to research that inflicted harm.

Exploitative?

Does this mean that the CII Project was exploitative, just as so much previous research has been?

On balance, I don't think so. Listen to Rebecca, an Aboriginal parent interviewee, who reports about the process:

> I like this ... talking about who we are, what we believe in, what we want for
> our kids. We should do more of this, without a cause. Kinda just sit around
> and share stories ... If we want to strengthen and save our heritage we need

to do these things and often ... [We need to] reach to family, gather, listen, and talk, share stories. Then the community will fall into place and time.

Denise, another Aboriginal mother, agrees:

I want to find a way for us to continue this work. I want to talk more about what we need to do, I feel like there is a light now at the end of the tunnel. *[pause, tears ...]* I am scared that we are gonna stop all of this, and it feels like we are so close to finding what is going on inside each of us.

Denise's remarks signal that the CII process sparked personal reflections and consciousness raising, which have significance for Aboriginal mothers far beyond the data. She and other individual study participants in one community have, therefore, organized opportunities to meet collectively. At their request, the CII Project committed resources to the initial meeting, which included a trained Indian residential school survivor group facilitator.

The desire to continue the CII process *as a programmatic intervention* to which Rebecca and Denise allude subsequently transformed the raison d'être of the CII Project. Aside from me, the executive team members are not working on academic papers. This had never been the plan. Rather, HIPPY staff wanted CII data to contribute to new program materials. But Denise, Rebecca, and others signalled that no new materials per se were needed. Rather, the CII team needed to enable others to facilitate the sort of conversations that our research interviews had started to generate.

Debbie, Tammy, and I set our minds to this task, in consultation with another excellent adult educator, Bonnie Soroke. Informed by my academic writing about the CII data, we selected excerpts from journals and interviews to create group facilitation strategies for others to follow. The result is that observations from CII participants are now starting points for conversations in which other Canadians, minority and majority, are asked to consider the relevance of the narrative insight to their own lives. Debbie and Tammy allocated $40,000 to develop and pilot these materials with Family Resource Programs across the country. Some of the ten community researchers were involved in training the group facilitators in other programs, providing HIPPY and Aboriginal HIPPY team members again with new employment roles and opportunities to travel. Debbie even attracted TeleVision Ontario to film one of the pilots in order to feature the group conversation as part of a documentary on public television, and an interactive website. In short, the other executive team members are taking the CII findings to communities across the country. And they are not waiting for or relying upon academic, peer-reviewed publications to justify their confidence in the data. Why would they? They're just sharing their own expertise.

Exploitation? If control over project funding is given to the community partner, I don't think exploitation is inherent to community-university collaborations, notwithstanding the examples to which some of my colleagues refer in this anthology. And I don't answer this way just because I'm a white boy blinded by my own privilege, or oblivious to the career advancement to which the unique CII data may contribute for me personally, even if the funding does not.

Consider what *we* achieved with the project. The funding helped secure the economic well-being of Aboriginal HIPPY and HIPPY for more than three years, programs that already existed because of the interest shown by minority community members. This security paved the way for both programs to divorce themselves from Simon Fraser University when they felt that their directors' contributions were not adequately valued. The project also paid wages, extended benefits, and provided more employment hours for ten women over three years. And their work in this project had heightened status. Aboriginal/HIPPY home visitors were experts. They were researchers. They are proud of these roles. And they increasingly see themselves as leaders in their communities.

Even parent participants gained financially. Each received $25 an hour for their time. While it only worked out to about $25 every six weeks, they told the home visitors they appreciated the money. Don't forget that HIPPY participants are low-income families. Plus, the mothers typically appreciated the process itself. Recall Rebecca and Denise, who want to continue the conversations that CII started for them. And it's not just the Aboriginal mothers. Hien, originally from Vietnam, comments:

> I think it [the research process] is very awesome, and it helps me to express my thoughts because there is nobody who has the time to ask me these kinds of questions.

No Hollywood Ending
Given its beginning, you might think this story has only happy endings. But we're not in Hollywood. While I stand firmly by the value of allocating

control for project finances to the community partners, two less than ideal outcomes are worth noting from the perspective of this white cow*boy* academic, above and beyond the risks for tenure and promotion.

First, the HIPPY and Aboriginal HIPPY plans to develop knowledge mobilization tools treated very casually the precision with which academics select their words. Initial drafts included text that essentialized cultural membership, was insufficiently critical about the gender division of labour, and even (unintentionally) stated that Aboriginal communities no longer suffer from the legacy of the Indian residential schools! These textual errors arose despite the fact that community team members knew our findings supported contrary conclusions. Even after community colleagues changed the text in the light of my editorial suggestions (which took a lot of time away from the academic writing I had planned to do), collaborators did not show sufficient care to ensure that the revised text was submitted for production. These examples highlight that academic-community collaborations may vulnerably position university partners because their findings, their voices, risk misrepresentation. In a business where the precision of ideas is paramount, this risk merits attention in future discussions about feminist collaborative methodologies.

The second troubling outcome occurred in our last full group research meeting. We asked, Where do we go from here? now that the data collection was complete and the community discussion guides were underway. The rest of the team decided their top priority was to produce a manual to conduct community research. The manual, they said, would empower communities with a research process that would not need university partners. They wanted my support.

This small white cow*boy* would not saddle his horse for their proposed trip.

In declining, I asked whether they wanted a manual to teach research, or a manual to teach community leadership. I'm convinced that my colleagues are wonderfully positioned to teach the latter. Debbie and Tammy were already community leaders when the project started. And my home visitor colleagues are increasingly confident to stand in front of groups, earning attention when they voice their opinions or encourage action. So why did they want to research, rather than lead?

If research is their priority, then academic expertise remains important. It doesn't have to be from an affluent white boy. But I am surprised that after three years together, my colleagues didn't think the academic expertise mattered.

In my view, my community colleagues, as great as they are, cannot yet research adequately on their own, so long as they want their experiential expertise to inform a body of knowledge that stretches beyond any individual's circumstances, or their findings to be taken seriously by people who value academic credentials. Their study design, implementation, and data analysis would not be of the same quality were it not informed by academic expertise. The challenges my community collaborators had when translating research findings into knowledge mobilization tools speaks to this issue.

I can hear you cringing. Maybe you are even thinking, "What a typical white man!" He's still privileging his own positivist expertise above that of others. How can he claim to do black feminist methodology or to understand indigenous epistemology? Why doesn't he exit the stage when others ask for the limelight?

Answer: Because the CII Project did not show that academics are redundant to community research. Rather, it showed that experiential and book-learned knowledge work in harmony. My community colleagues may not need a conductor. But singing a cappella is much more difficult than performing with a band. It's not impossible. But it takes a lot of practice.

There is another reason I declined, although I choose these final words carefully so I don't imply that minority communities need outsiders for research support.

If less privileged communities grow content to research apart from academics, they risk privatizing responsibility for social change. This does not mean that communities need academic permission to ask questions or provide answers, especially not from white boys like me. But encouraging them to ask and answer without university support may disoblige some who are privileged from facilitating other people telling their stories, sharing their expertise.

To be sure, any story about white cow*boys* doing black feminist community research guided by Indian narratives will be fraught with ethical tensions. But if white boys narrate only their "own" stories for fear of being tangled by these tensions, they ignore that they are systemically empowered to command attention for voices they respect. They forgo opportunities to subvert their unearned privilege.

ACKNOWLEDGMENTS
The Care, Identity, and Inclusion Project provides the context for the methodological reflections I share about feminist community-based research in this chapter. Community collaborators in the Aboriginal HIPPY and HIPPY programs tell

invaluable stories about the political, cultural, and religious significance of care-giving for identity. Their stories merit greater attention.

In telling this methodological story, I am indebted to the book's other contributors for insightful feedback that they provided about earlier drafts. Special thanks are owed to Joan Anderson, Jane Pulkingham, Shawna Butterwick, Silvia Vilches, Colleen Reid, and Wendy Frisby.

REFERENCES

Chrisjohn, Roland, and Sherri Young. 2006. *The Circle Game: Shadows and Substance in the Indian Residential School Experience in Canada.* 2nd ed. Penticton, BC: Theytus Books.

Collins, Patricia Hill. 1991. *Black Feminist Thought: Knowledge, Consciousness, and the Politics of Empowerment.* New York and London: Routledge.

–. 1994. "Shifting the Center: Race, Class, and Feminist Theorizing about Motherhood." In E.N. Glenn, G. Chang, and L.R. Forcey, eds., *Mothering: Ideology, Experience, and Agency,* 45-66. New York: Routledge.

Dua, Enakshi. 1999. "Beyond Diversity: Exploring the Ways in Which the Discourse of Race Has Shaped the Institution of the Nuclear Family." In E. Dua and A. Robertson, eds., *Scratching the Surface: Canadian Anti-Racist Feminist Thought,* 237-60. Toronto: Women's Press.

Kershaw, Paul. 2005. *Carefair: Rethinking the Responsibilities and Rights of Citizenship.* Vancouver: UBC Press.

King, Thomas. 2003. *The Truth about Stories: A Native Narrative.* Toronto: House of Anansi.

Roberts, Dorothy E. 1995. "Racism and Patriarchy in the Meaning of Motherhood." In M.A. Fineman and I. Karpin, eds., *Mothers in Law: Feminist Theory and the Legal Regulation of Motherhood,* 224-49. New York: Columbia University Press.

Simien, Evelyn M. 2007. "Doing Intersectionality Research: From Conceptual Issues to Practical Examples." *Politics and Gender* 3 (2): 264-71.

Trevithick, Scott. 1998. "Native Residential Schooling in Canada: A Review of the Literature." *Canadian Journal of Native Studies* 28(1): 49-86.

UNICEF. 2008. "The Child Care Transition: A League Table of Early Childhood Education and Care in Economically Advanced Countries." In *Innocenti Report Card 8.* Florence: UNICEF Innocenti Research Centre. http://www.unicef.ca/portal/Secure/Community/502/WCM/HELP/take_action/Advocacy/rc8.pdf.

Visweswaran, Kamala. 1994. *Fictions of Feminist Ethnography.* Minneapolis: University of Minnesota Press.

Wolf, Diane. 1996. *Feminist Dilemmas in Fieldwork.* Boulder, CO: Westview Press.

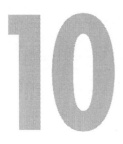

Inside and Outside of the Gates
Transforming Relationships through Research

RUTH ELWOOD MARTIN, KELLY MURPHY,
AND MARLA J. BUCHANAN

From Kelly's field notes:
A provincial prison is not the typical place that one would
anticipate a career move; nor did I know back in 2005, as I
sat waiting to see the prison doctor, that in four years' time
we would be working together on a research project outside
of the gates.

How are research relationships reconstituted from the traditional dichotomy of researcher/subject within a prison research project that values collaborative participation, authentic relationships, community, reflexivity, transparency, and transformation?

In this chapter, Ruth and Kelly use their field notes, journal entries, and academic writing to reflect upon their research relationships within three phases of a prison-based collaborative participatory action research project. Marla facilitates an analysis of their experiences from the position of feminist methodologist.

Traditional medical research positions Ruth as the principal investigator conducting research inside a women's correctional facility and Kelly as the inmate prison subject. Within traditional medical practice, Ruth is defined as a prison family physician and Kelly a prison patient. Each of these subject positions have power differentials, and the structure of their roles already exists before the research project begins.

In this chapter, we show how community-based participatory research processes necessitated a shift in Kelly's and Ruth's power differentials; indeed, we describe how community-based participatory research processes are possible only when pre-existing power differentials do transform. In this chapter, we interweave our shifting positions to demonstrate the struggles in participatory action research, and we reflect upon our practices and conversations as a way of understanding the knowledge produced in this project.

We define participatory action research using McTaggart's description (1991, 171-72):

> Authentic participation in research means sharing in the way research is conceptualized, practiced, and brought to bear on the life-world. It means ownership – responsible agency in the production of knowledge and the improvement of practice ... In participatory action research the real test is that people are actually conducting the research for themselves and reflecting on its nature ... individuals and groups agree to work together to change themselves, individually and collectively. Their interests are joined by an agreed thematic concern.

We ask, How have we been transformed or emancipated through participation in this project? As Wadsworth (1998) states about the process of participatory action research: "Change does not happen at the 'end' – it happens throughout."

Phase I – Researching inside Prison

Ruth

I have worked part-time as a physician in the medical clinics of provincial prisons since 1994. It's as if I am visiting another planet, passing through those gates. I'm experiencing another world and learning from the people in it.

The prison is a minimum/medium security women's correctional facility in a western province in Canada. In five cottage-style living units, it housed approximately 120 women, each of whom had an average stay of sixty days; some of the women were still awaiting trial. Approximately 1,600 women revolved through the provincial correctional system per year, with a disproportionately high number of Aboriginal women. Women in prison have poorer health, with a higher prevalence of HIV infection, hepatitis C, cervical dysplasia, and psychiatric illness than the general population. The majority of women with short prison sentences in Canada are imprisoned because of illegal activities stemming from drug and/or alcohol misuse.

We conducted initial exploratory work with individual and group interviews of incarcerated women and prison staff to pose two questions: What would participatory action health research look like in prison? What health issues would you like to see prison-based participatory action research address? Subsequently, we invited all women in prison, prison staff and management, and academic researchers to attend a day-long face-to-face meeting in the prison gym. At the meeting, we hoped to share the findings from the exploratory work, brainstorm ideas for potential participatory health research, and invite women and prison staff to assist in writing a funding proposal.

The prison Aboriginal Elder suggested that we open the meeting with a prayer and invited the chaplain to do so conjointly with her. Everyone stood in a large circle and held hands – incarcerated women, correctional centre staff, and academic researchers. In the centre of the circle, the Elder said a prayer in Cree and then translated it into English. The prison chaplain then said a prayer in English.

We then presented the themes that had emerged from the exploratory work. Following this, an open microphone session enabled all women, correctional staff, and academic researchers to contribute. During this process, the Elder assisted with fostering respectful participation: if an individual had the microphone, they were to be the only one talking. During the process, participants voiced and agreed on five values: (1) transparency of all information; (2) break the code of silence; (3) respect for diversity – listen and be heard; (4) build on strengths; and (5) all who wish to be involved in the research process may be involved.

Later, I would tell my friends and colleagues that, short of birthing my kids and getting married, this day, the day of the prison health research forum, 14 October 2005, ranked up there for me in terms of life-changing moments. There I was, prison physician for years, working in the prison clinic and encountering women only in the confines of the clinical examining room, and here I was in the gym facilitating a venture that was moving us all into the unknown – inmates, correctional officers, wardens, health care staff – working on it together. The day seemed almost magical. The hope in the gym was almost palpable.

Kelly

It's difficult to put into words what it felt like to have had the opportunity to be in that first forum. It was presented to a hundred or so inmates that we had an ability to bring about change in the health of incarcerated women; now and in the future. The closest I can get to describing it is "magical," thrilling, and now in hindsight, miraculous.

Awestruck, I was, as Dr. Martin and her colleagues addressed the room full of broken women about how we could come together, as women, and work on ways to get our lives back. We listened to her tell us:

> Over the years, I have known many of you as patients. I have witnessed you cycle in and out, in and out, suffering from a multitude of health problems. I have listened to your stories of one hurdle after another preventing you from leading healthy lives, and I have wept with you. I have ached with the unanswered question of What can be done to improve the health of women in prison? I have led several traditional research projects looking at one or another aspect of that question.
>
> In the spring of 2005, while I was studying an online Action Research course, I had an "Aha!" moment – a light bulb experience. What would happen if women in prison could research their own health issues? What would a collaborative research project, a project grounded in the women's lived experience, tell us about their health concerns? I realized that this was the type of research we should be doing in prison.

We broke into smaller groups in the afternoon so that we could brainstorm the different topics that had been brought to the table that morning.

I don't think that there were many women sleeping that night in the camp; all pumped up on adrenaline and empowerment, many of us anticipating the meeting that was called into action for the following day for those that would want to participate on the research project. There is nothing more gratifying to me than the look of hope in a woman's eyes.

Ruth

The next morning, twenty-seven women inmates arrived in the gym to help us to write the funding application for a prison community-based participatory health research project. The following week, the women asked the warden if she would make the "research team" a prison work placement, similar to other prison work placements such as laundry and cleaning. Two weeks later, when we submitted the funding application, the women asked if they might continue their research project work (while we waited for the funding to arrive), as the work had become meaningful for them.

At that time we had no funding and, therefore, no research support staff. The woman offered to do the research themselves. "We don't need funding," they explained; they had lots of time on their hands and they wanted to learn. The serendipity of the lack of funding meant that incarcerated women guided every aspect of the research process *themselves*. Several of the academic members on the team volunteered to visit the prison to facilitate research skill-building workshops for the women. For myself, I decided to "do research" with the women in the prison research room on Mondays and to "do medicine" in the prison clinic on Tuesdays. I would shift between the two roles, on Mondays as "Dr. Ruth the researcher" and on Tuesdays as "Dr. Martin the prison doctor." The women seemed to accept this.

Up to fifteen women met daily on the prison participatory health research team – some women stayed on the team for one or two weeks, others for several months – and, over the next twenty-two months, almost two hundred women became members of the research team. The women developed an orientation package for new members, which included several written exercises – a new members' survey, a paragraph of passion exercise, and a drug of choice survey. They developed a daily routine for themselves that included a devotional reading and angel cards. Activities included educational presentations created and given by the women on the prison research team (including hosting prison health research forums to which they invited academic researchers, community agencies, funders, and policy makers; developing a library of health education PowerPoint presentations; and visiting a local high school to educate and share their stories about alcohol and drug use); surveys created and conducted by women on the research team; interventions initiated by women on the prison research team (including hosting participatory qualitative analysis workshops, writing workshops, and research discussions with academic researchers; and creating a Web page to host project and community information for women leaving prison); and interventions initiated by prison staff.

Kelly

Respect was evident for the most part with the women who participated on the research team inside. When a group of women get together, a group of survivors that is, there seems to be camaraderie, which oversees ego and pride. A natural pecking order, kind of like on the street, we all assume our roles and functions within the group, and this all seems to happen quite naturally.

We have our own community that started from the outside, in the life of crime, which moves to the inside and determines who you are. Your character and how you conducted yourself determine the level of respect that you would receive once you land in prison.

I am not sure if the same respect exists for the women that came in from the outside. Sure, we were polite and minded our manners, so to speak, but if you aren't from jail, you just aren't one of us. We would respect the outsiders because we had to, we were in jail after all, and besides it was easier to simulate respect in order to get what we wanted. Conformity, isn't that what it's called?

Simply put, I think that respect is something that needs to be earned. Inside prison we have worked out how that respect is to be established. If you come from the outside, there is always an order of things. If you are from the outside and you are not a criminal, then how can you fit into the "order of things"? There will always be an "us and them" attitude if one is not imprisoned, within the gates, that is.

Ruth
I found that I began to enjoy my days in the research room more than my days in the clinic – the research days became a bit like "kitchen table wisdom" over cups of tea, as the women talked about what they were interested in – whatever topic they were researching at the time. It felt a more meaningful use of my time. At times I felt like a mother, at times like a mentor, at times a big sister, at times a research expert, at times a translator of medical information. But, so many days, I felt like the learner.

My favourite part of the day was joining in the angel cards routine, because this exercise seemed to root us together in something bigger than what we might accomplish on our own. And, I was often moved to awe, humbled, as I listened to their spiritual journeys, by the depth of their understanding and their resilience.

From the Transcript of the Inmate Research Team Morning Meeting, 18 November 2005

"Angel Cards"

Woman #1
Ok, good morning everybody. I'll explain the little cards that we have. Just like to welcome our guests that we have here today. Welcome. We have a lot of new girls here today. So, first of all, we always start our meeting with a little prayer, and then after that we're going to do the words we picked out. So, we're just going to go around the room with everybody and, depending

on the word that you have, explain what that means to you and how you feel today, ok? ... so, we just talk with each other and tell each other how we feel, because we're all working together as a team to do this research. My word of the day is *overcome*. Wow, that's a big word. This is the first time I've ever been separated from my son, who's going to be thirteen on the twenty-fifth of this month. So, I've learnt to overcome my past life and realize the mistakes that I have done, because my heart was broken when I first came in. I'm overcoming my obstacles, I'm fighting every one of them, and this program and this research just fills me every day. I'm just go, go, go every day, um, and work till, like, seven o'clock every night.

Woman #2
My word's *intuition*. Intuition to me means that we have a voice inside us, a small voice, sometimes hard to listen to, but it's there, and we should be aware, and we should listen to it.

Woman #3
My word is *forgiveness,* and what that means to me is that you have to forgive yourself before you can forgive anybody else. And I'm just great. I got some exciting news, um, I wrote an article for our joint effort newsletter. It's actually, it's a woman's magazine; it's called the "Word of Op," and they are publishing an article about our [prison research] forum. And they asked me to write more, they asked me to keep, so I'll just ...

Woman #4
My word is *energy,* and I just think that that means that I probably, I don't know, I have to be aware of my energy and the way that other people's energy effects me. Can't say I'm fantastic, but I'm not. But I have ... yeah, today is the anniversary of, like, it's my second kid's thirteenth birthday, and it's seven years ago today that I lost my four kids. So much has happened to me. I guess if I pull that word up, I have to be aware of that energy that I put out there, so I'm trying to go with that. Thanks.

Kelly
She didn't actually leave her bag sitting there, unattended in a room of convicted criminals? I remember feeling somewhat protective over Dr. Martin's bag at the same time, thinking, "What is in the bag, and do I have enough time to snoop through it?" I saw some of the other girls in the room staring at the bag. Were they contemplating the same things as I was? Were my thoughts infectious? Was I contaminating them with my thoughts, or were

they polluting me with theirs? Here I was in a place where my past was trying to infiltrate the present, and I had declared to myself and others that I was going to make a change. But what if one of the other girls caught me in my altruistic mindset? I just wouldn't be cool. Then, what would happen with the rest of my stay at "camp cupcake"? It was one of those defining moments, where the decision I was making in the present would shape my future; just do the next right thing. She left with her bag intact that day, and me, I left prison with integrity – a renewed aspect of character that had been expressionless for far too long.

Ruth

I remember the day that the women of the prison research team were invited to talk to the local high school about the harmful effects of drug and alcohol use. They were allowed to pick street clothes from the prison thrift store supplies. They also picked out jeans for me and the prison recreation therapist, so that the teenagers might not be able to distinguish the recreation therapist and prison physician from the women on the research team. When nine women walked out in single file onto the high school stage, in a line, to the sound of the Red Hot Chili Peppers, and the applause of about 150 Grade 11 students, I felt as if my heart would burst.

Our Reflections on Participatory Research

The ceremonial beginning of this project placed us on a path that honoured collaboration, community, and spiritual connection.

As Ruth describes her dual roles, we can see how ethics, power, and knowledge shift in relation to the positions that she takes up. As she works in her role as prison researcher on a project investigating incarcerated women's health concerns, she cannot pretend not to know the women's medical histories. She has insider knowledge that others do not have. In her conscious efforts to bracket insider medical health knowledge, she engages in her research work with "new eyes," open to new knowledge of health concerns framed from the ground up. She has to be vigilant of research ethics, dual relationships, and boundary violations in this research project in addition to surveilling how she frames the knowledge that she generates, that is, asking questions such as: Whose knowledge is this? Who benefits from this knowledge? Who is at risk if we generate this knowledge?

As Ruth and Kelly reflect on the early stages of the research project, their multiple roles and subjectivities point to the ways in which they both experience challenges and possibilities. They engage in the discourse of prison research, wearing different uniforms, using different language, holding different positions, and working through the multiple hierarchies inherent in research relationships. How can they get beyond these borders? How can they build the trust needed to reconfigure insider/outsider distinctions? Is it even possible?

In the final paragraph, we see the power of the material world as possibly separating Kelly and Ruth as collaborators in the project. The clothing, a material distinction, has the capacity to separate, creating "Otherness." The prison researchers, seeking a level ground from which to present their work demonstrates the reflexivity inherent in our PAR process and the trust that was being built on the research team.

Phase 2 – Power Plays

Ruth

This writing becomes a venue for me to debrief and to pull it all together in my head, in a way that I haven't done before now. Women in prison started to face a stream of continuous hurdles, which thwarted their full engagement in participatory health and education research. It began in February 2007, when the warden asked the women not to conduct their peer survey of "mother and child separation" because of concerns that the survey itself might be harmful and might trigger negative thoughts and behaviour among women inside prison. The survey had been designed and piloted by women of the prison research team and had received full university research ethics board approval. By that date, the women had already successfully conducted approximately ten peer surveys inside prison.

We were then told that women in prison were no longer allowed to "co-author" research articles, publications, or conference presentations – their names needed to be protected from the public. In the spring of 2007, I was told to cease a publication of an intended medical journal article, for which we were then reviewing the journal galley proofs, because several inmates were co-authors of the article.

Women of the prison health research team met together to formulate their response to Corrections Branch, as follows:

> We, women of the Prison Health Research Team, are proud of our work. We feel that all the research work that we do brings us credibility. It helps us to rehabilitate.

Students studying at university use their names on their writing, PowerPoint creations, and publications, and we wish to do the same. Our research work is our achievement and our voice: it describes what we are doing; it records what we are doing. It doesn't make sense that anyone else is acknowledged for the work that we have done. We are damn proud of our work and we wish to be recognized. In addition, if we want to find employment in a related field (e.g., journalism, writing, health research) then we need these publications and presentations for our resumes.

Just because we're inmates we're not hidden away. Anyone could find our names on the Internet through court proceedings. We can't hide our identities. Any job that we apply for in the future will recognize that we were inmates, because we have a criminal record. In addition, the media often portrays us, using our full names, by inaccurate and negative descriptions, about which we have no choice. The Women's Prison Health Research Team provides us with the opportunity to contribute positively to society and to be acknowledged for doing so.

We recognize that some time later (months, years) our views may have changed from what we said publicly while we were members of the Prison Health Research Team. But this is growth; it happens to the best of authors or public speakers.

The warden told me to disconnect the project Web page from the Internet until "Branch approval" was obtained. I asked how one obtains "Branch approval," but I received no information about how to acquire it. Women in prison were then refused permission for future temporary absences to give presentations at community conferences or lectures. For example, women in prison were told they could not present at local high schools or conferences. Women in prison were told to stop creating surveys and to discontinue hosting or organizing all health and research prison forums for the prison community and/or outside guests.

Once they were told they could not create any more surveys, and their stationery supplies were curtailed, the women developed an underground method for doing surveys. For example, the women created a survey by writing their survey questions on small pieces of scrap paper. They would take turns sitting outside on the grass, quietly asking their questions of their living unit peers about exercise and nutrition and writing the responses down verbatim. Word spread, and women gathered, clandestinely, to take their turn at completing the survey orally. Women on the research team computed the survey percentages by hand, adding the responses manually on recycled paper.

Previously, I had copied all my prison-related research e-mails to both the warden and research director, as a way of communicating all the project details to them. Now, a Participatory Action Research Supervisory Committee was to oversee all aspects of the research project, and it would include the current warden, the research director, the medical director, the mental health director, and the incoming prison warden. I was asked to copy *all* my research correspondence, e-mails, and writings to *all* members of this committee. The PAR Supervisory Committee would have monthly tele-conference call meetings to decide which research activities they would permit. Activities would be approved by the committee, if the women on the research team submitted a prior proposal to the supervisory committee. The committee held monthly teleconferences for two months, then summer meetings were cancelled; no subsequent meetings were scheduled.

In effect, the creation of this committee paralyzed the activities of the women's prison participatory research project. For example, women wrote a proposal to convert their PowerPoint presentations into electronic interactive modules for the computers on the prison living units. The committee gave them absolutely no feedback for this proposal; members of the committee did not reply to my e-mails. It was heartbreaking – I felt powerless.

In the fall, the warden phoned me to explain that we no longer had "Branch approval" to proceed with our resubmission of the Canadian Institutes of Health Research (CIHR) operating grant. I responded that I must meet face to face with Corrections Branch personnel, in order to talk through this decision (and others), in an effort to arrive at mutual understanding and collaboration. I booked to fly to Branch Headquarters to meet with them; when my flight was cancelled because of fog, we rescheduled for the following month. One evening, a corrections officer called together the women in prison on the research team. She informed them that, as of the following week, there would no longer be a "research project" in the prison. The women were to clean out their research room and would be assigned to different work placement jobs. The women's immediate reaction was that they must have done something terribly wrong to result in cancellation of the research team. They wondered if I had authorized the dissolution of the research team.

In the turmoil of "How should we respond?" it is hard to know which response will effect the most beneficial long-term results. At a personal level, one can get angry and write protest letters and ranting e-mails. We can also mobilize that response collectively. I delayed my scheduled vacation, visited the prison, and invited women to come together for an ad hoc debriefing evening meeting in the "research room." Approximately thirty women came; each woman reacting differently to the disbandment of the research team. Many women were in tears. Many were angry. A high-profile incarcerated environmentalist and activist encouraged women to strike and to refuse to work inside prison. Some women talked about writing letters to the media. Gradually, I sensed passive, hopeless, resignation descend over the group.

When I returned from my holiday, I received a letter from Corrections Branch, which stated:

> [We] regret to inform you that the Corrections Branch can no longer support the participatory action research at the _____ Correctional Centre for Women.
>
> The ongoing challenges with scope, definition and direction of the project, unsecured resources, operational and administrative demands, and a lack of clear policy and program benefit, have rendered this project unsustainable for the Branch.
>
> All activity related to this research must now cease (including solicitations for offender participation, ongoing PAR communications with ____ staff, etc).
>
> As per s. 16 of the research agreement, all hard copy materials gathered for conducting this research that contain any personal information on offenders at _____ (e.g., surveys, data, informed consent forms, etc.) in your possession or under your purview, must be shredded or returned to Corrections headquarters as soon as possible. All electronic copies of these materials must be deleted from your computer(s) and those of associated researchers participating in this project.
>
> We will require written notice that you have complied with this aspect of the research agreement no later than October 15, 2007.

I was devastated. I felt that I had let the women in prison down. I wondered what I might have done differently, to prevent the shutting down of this project. I asked university lawyers for advice. They advised me to cancel my previously scheduled meeting with Corrections Branch and, instead, to write a letter. I did this, and I received no reply to my letter.

In my confusion and anxiety during the events leading up to receipt of the letter, my major concern had been to be able to preserve doing some semblance of participatory health research within the prison, for the sake of the women involved. As time went on, it became apparent to me that it was untenable to continue conducting participatory research under a changing prison milieu, including a new prison warden who was not supportive of the project.

Later, as I reflected, I came to realize that community-based participatory research must build on shared values and on a continual process of creating partnerships – where equal voices are respected – as we had earlier articulated in our five-year research agreement, which Corrections Branch signed and agreed to with us in March 2006. If we are ever to re-establish participatory health research inside prison, we would first need to reaffirm these guiding values for the project.

Hence, after two years of the five-year project, the Corrections Branch stated that they would no longer permit the prison participatory research project to continue. Other initiatives, which the warden had also introduced, aligned with a vision of a therapeutic prison community, were similarly cancelled; the warden was subsequently asked to leave the post.

Our Reflections on Participatory Research in Phase 2

As feminist researchers we need to ask how an institution that gave consent for a research project can withdraw the individual consent of women who voluntarily and knowingly gave their own consent? It is a breach of ethics, to say the least, but is it legal to withdraw the consent of another without dialogue or avenues to contest the involuntary withdrawal of another? The prison administrators, as the official gatekeepers, had the power to withdraw and curtail practices within their gates. Their actions were not only patronizing, but can be viewed as institutional violence. We ask: What was the threat? What were the risks to the prison administration and staff? What politics were taking place behind closed doors? Their silence is deafening. As Michelle Fine and Maria Elena Torre note in their four-year study on the impact of providing college in prison (2004, 27),

> Prison administrators were and remain the gatekeepers to changes in policy and practice. PAR relies on co-researchers, many of whom are profound critics, a number of whom are most vulnerable. Those who dare to speak from within run an enormous risk of retribution. Therein lies the danger of *speaking*.

The prison research project went underground. These acts of resistance are evidence of the women's self-empowerment, their commitment to their own health, and their struggle with relations of power. Their knowledge would not be silenced. Their passion was tenable.

Fine and Torre point out that "the dominant story told about institutional life is but one story and typically told from the 'top,' and that critical understandings of power and inequity while usually buried, are essential to the democratic resuscitation of public institutions" (2004, 18). What is missing in Ruth's account of the events that took place is a clearer or transparent understanding about how the knowledge being produced threatened the prison system or put anyone at risk. The silence on the part of the prison is an act of aggression, and its oppressive impact on the lives of the women in prison, on both the researchers and their peers, and on the academic researchers on the outside, had real effects.

The women in prison went underground and retaliated with their own brand of clandestine survey research design. The academic researchers consulted with lawyers and research boards to obtain advice on how to proceed with the research. The retribution from the prison system illustrates the power/knowledge dynamics that get played out when those in authority make decisions that are not collaborative or consultative. Knowledge in this illustration rests solely with the privileges of institutional power: "PAR designs are not only dedicated to revealing the gross effects of institutional inequity on those deprived; they can also reveal how institutions produce and protect privilege" (Fine and Torre 2004, 23).

Phase 3: Outside the Gates

Ruth

We had always encouraged women to come and work with the research team at our university following their release from prison, but none had. In August 2007, as one woman was preparing for her release, I said, "Kelly, if you would like to come and volunteer on the research team, please do get in touch with us." She did.

So, in the serendipity of the unfolding of events, our community focus increased as the prison focus was being decreased. Through Kelly, other women who have been released from prison have joined the participatory research project Women In2 Healing, which is focused on the health and educational goals of women who leave prison.

Kelly

I think that it's always a miracle when we can organize women to meet on the outside who had spent time with each other inside of prison. Some of these women I have known for many years, way back into the days of drugs and crime, and some I know from prison. I can't begin to describe the joy that I experience when I look at how these women are now "doing life" instead of "doing time." It is particularly heart-warming to watch the young women with their children. When I observe these women, I am in awe over the love that they have for their children, and I wonder what was the catalyst that motivated the change in their lives? For each woman it is different, but what I do know is that we can't do it alone. What a blessing, to have the opportunity to hear their stories and to be present in their journey through this participatory research project.

It was a long trip that Saturday morning, and as usual we were late; it is often that way with our research group. We forgot the directions, and the anxiety was accelerating (so was Dr. Martin's foot on the gas pedal) as we approached the Coffee House.

We weren't certain as to how many of the invitees from the released women would actually attend. There were twenty-three confirmed women; however, past events had shown that this number would dwindle as the day finally arrived.

The research team that had originated inside the gates of the prison, and is currently outside the gates within the community, had been busy trying to get released women together. It was in the agenda that we would to try to come up with some ideas for a new name for the project and a logo for our Web page, do some Christmas art, discuss life: many of us hadn't seen each other since we were inside the gates. So, the anticipation was high, as we gathered in the boardroom, all dressed in our "Sunday best." At this point I would like to make mention of all the attendees; however, I hesitate to do so in case I leave someone out. I will say that we had fourteen women who had formerly been incarcerated. There were the academics and our mentors who have been with us since the beginning of the project. Two of the women even brought their little babies, and one girl brought her sister and her sister's baby. It was a full room, especially when all the babies were crying at once.

If you can, picture this among twenty different women, from different backgrounds, various ethnicities; each exclusive in our own way. Where we started was confined in cells, all of us imprisoned in our hell, and now here we were on the other side: no longer victims of our circumstances but women of power and authority over our own lives. Each one of us is unique in understanding freedom as our own experience. It was awe-inspiring and life-changing for myself, and I felt so blessed to have the opportunity to be there.

Ruth

During an International Primary Care Research Conference, as I listened to the presentations of women who are engaged in this project, I realized that they wish to learn a new and different way of responding. They told me that it is easy for them to respond in anger, negativity, or with passive resignation (and/or internal anger), because this is how they are used to responding. However, they told me that this project provided them with opportunities to learn how to respond differently to adverse circumstances.

With time, I will seek to re-establish communication with Corrections Branch. I now have a better understanding of the key players and whom to approach. I now know the importance of creating powerful allies and advocates within the political field. I now see that Corrections Branch will not readily approve a "doing good work" health research project that empowers women in prison, because it threatens their overall mandate and "control system." I will continue to strive for policy changes whereby prisons for women incorporate increased participatory approaches to health and education, so that prisons become places of healing for women instead of places of punishment.

Kelly

As we gathered around the pretentious boardroom table, I contemplate the anxiety that I consistently encounter, before, during, and after these monthly meetings of the co-investigators. It has occurred to me that it might be the setting, the boardroom, and the vast distance around the table. Or could it be the name "co-investigators"? Just that word makes me want to hire a lawyer. My thoughts are wandering, and I am visualizing a different meeting place. The local pub, perhaps, or the back of a coffee house; the smell of fresh ground beans and baked goods. What would the atmosphere feel like then? Would there be the obvious distinction between academics, peer researchers, and project staff? Yes, I can envision it now, everyone dressed in jeans, t-shirts, and flip flops; many of the academics looking like a throw-back from the '60s. One would not be able to differentiate between PHD, CSC, MA, or MLA; in fact, letters would be of no concern. Bumptious academics would unify with the struggling students (the peer researchers) in a meaningful way that emanates "participatory." That is not to say that this is not happening; it's just that there is tension, and that is evident and really uncomfortable to me. Now keep in mind that this is my perspective, my processing of an environment that is still quite foreign to me. I consider that if I can't manage to navigate through two hours a month of seeming "pleasantries and play acting," then how will I ever manoeuvre through the ranks of UBC academia?

I bring myself back to the room in mid-conversation to a language that is completely alien to me. SPSS, SAQ, group force method, and, oh, the ever-so-popular "psychometric properties." With notable frustration in my voice, I kindly interrupt the speaker, so that the terms being used might be clarified. As my frustration continued to escalate, I struggled to stay in the room, to remain cognitively present. My thoughts kept wandering to the Women In2 Healing members (WitH), the previous research project that started inside prison, and wondering how they were digesting all of this "over the top" language. Maybe I was just trying to caretake their feelings, being a recovering co-dependant and all. Labels, shit!

As I sit here writing, I realize that my outlook might appear somewhat cynical; be that as it may, it is my process. I wasn't entirely certain as to what was transpiring for the other members of WitH, until a door was opened into the conversation regarding "values" of the project. I have never been a person who could just sit back and allow the elephant to tromp around the room without naming it. I felt the need to speak something, anything, in order to dispel the obvious tension. But what, what was I going to say that wouldn't make me look like an idiot? As I sat there praying, asking God to provide an opening, my will took over. Who cares? This is participatory, and sometimes I forget that. There isn't such a thing as a wrong way of approaching process. And, more than anything, I wanted the other women to feel safe to speak out also; to come forward, if they felt the need to do so. I risk my face for the sake of the others; after all, it is only false pride and ego. It wouldn't be the first time in my life I appeared a fool, and after all, who was I judging here but myself? "Stop it, step up, step out!"

In validating my process, a conversation of authenticity broke out; the real deal. Unfortunately, it was so late into the meeting; it felt somewhat restrained from its full potential. It was, however, a beginning. As I sat, I thought about what a meeting might have looked like if WitH had the opportunity to actually "process" for an hour? Would it bridge the gap of tension? Or is the tension only mine?

Ruth

These days, I am so much more aware of the power of language, everyday words in medicine that I never previously questioned.

Kelly

Today, Nancy and I had our first interview appointment booked at the Downtown Eastside. I don't think I slept very well the night before in anticipation of what was to be. Although I have experienced a renewing of the mind when it comes to addiction, I think that still I get anxious when it comes to entering the environment. This is good information to have when we think about the potential harm that could be caused if we send "recovering" peer researchers into the field.

So, we headed down early with our baseline interviews, confidentiality forms, and the digital recorder. We got there about fifteen minutes early, only to be bombarded by a bunch of women asking us if "we were the women that were doing the survey." Instantly, I felt overwhelmed, and my crowd-control skills came into play. Clearly, we had to question each woman to discover when it was that she had actually been released from prison, and after the barrage we were left with five women who met the criteria of having been released within a week. Now, I'm not sure if all these women were telling the truth or not, and I really only recognized two of them from my past visits to prison. But what are we to do? We are going to have to come up with a tactic as to how to sift through to the truth. I think to inquire as to when they were actually released as opposed to "Were you released within the last week?"

I have to say that it was an emotionally exhausting experience. I am comforted to know that I haven't become apathetic to the lives of women that are entrenched downtown. I look and see myself in their lives and know that it is that close if I choose to make different choices. So, how do I help? We are not a resource for women who need help, and quite frankly, from the women that I spoke to, they are aware of the resources downtown, and it would appear that they utilize them frequently. Comfort, care, and concern are what I can offer. My last interview stated that I gave her hope and that I was a "beacon of light." It was because we had a personal relationship inside the gates of prison that there was a sense of trust. I had an epiphany as to why we are women who are connecting with each other.

Conversation, Ruth and Kelly, May 2009

Ruth: When we started off inside prison, we would not have thought that this would be possible.
Kelly: Who would?
Ruth: I now get to walk with you in your life outside prison.
Kelly: The other day, when we were sitting around, all of a sudden I looked at you (I think we were talking about age), and I realized that I have been present for three of your birthdays; and you have been present for one of mine, and you came to my confirmation and now, here, today, at my church. And it made me start thinking about all the important milestones in our lives and how this relationship from inside prison has moved to the outside, and we're celebrating life together. It's like we're best friends. We don't talk on the phone every day, right – you aren't my best friend in that sense – but it's a heart connection. I know that if I needed you, I could pick up the phone and you would be there in a minute. And, also, because we have a common ground in several areas – prison, research work, being a mother – a spiritual connection. But in these intimate moments, there's that relationship and that heart connection and that trust. It's a level of trust and integrity.

Our Reflections

Moving from inside to outside, changing contexts have had significant implications for the new research team. Insider/outsider status has changed, and the "community of academia" is contrasted to the "community inside prison." Contexts matter, and the discourses within these contexts have real effects on practices such as language usage, values, sense of self as a researcher, and other research actions (such as sitting around a board table in a medical setting). As Kelly notes, language usage matters. In her example it separates and creates hierarchies of knowledge/power. It affects research relationships – are we being transparent, collaborative, authentic in our interactions?

Our ability to remain critically reflexive about our practices of privilege is our only recourse to equitable research relationships and the establishment of community.

Kelly's struggle also parallels, to some degree, the struggles women have transitioning from prison to the "outside." As her context changes, her life also changes. As Ruth moves from prison physician to the principal investigator in an academic setting, her context also changes and has challenges that need to be recognized. Kelly's personal story is commensurate with the research she is conducting. Her insider knowledge is significant to this project, but we must also support Kelly in ways that promote the community-based participatory values that we uphold. We cannot lose sight of who we share the table with in this research project.

Conclusions: Transforming Relationships through Research

At the beginning of this chapter, we asked, How are research relationships reconstituted from the traditional dichotomy of researcher/subject within a prison research project that valued collaborative participation, authentic relationships, community, reflexivity, transparency, and transformation? Over the two separate phases of the research, inside and outside prison, we believed that the values of our research team members were upheld. We worked at building research relationships that honoured mutuality, respect, trust, and honesty. However, we were remiss in not continually confirming congruency between our research team's values and the values of our stakeholders within the prison setting. There were many obstacles and miscommunications regarding our conduct in establishing participatory research within prison. However, many lessons were learned that will facilitate future participatory research in these contexts. Several questions were raised that need to be addressed before engaging in future prison research.

Reflections of Institutional Power

Trust among stakeholders, political naïveté on the part of the research team, and inequitable relations of power were pitfalls that undermined our participatory aims in conducting prison research. We also believe that political changes at the federal level with a new government that is "tough on crime," and changes within the prison setting with a new warden, influenced the changes that occurred within our research relationships. We need to be wary of privilege and power and critically reflect on whose authority or privilege determines the next steps in participatory research. Do those in authority share our research values? Do we pose a threat to their institutional power? What are the politics of knowledge at play in our research acts? In future research, we will need to establish regular and ongoing communication efforts/strategies to keep gatekeepers informed of our research progress in order to diminish institutional barriers as the research unfolds. We need to keep tabs on relations of power, voice, authority, and privilege in our future research endeavours.

Reflections on Participation and Collaboration

Important issues to discern in prison research concern participation and collaboration. Given the inequity on issues of power, freedom, and access, several questions arise that need to be addressed in future research: Who decides who participates, and with what contributions and roles? Is participation transparent? Is participation accessible, equitable, or contingent? Are efforts in research collaboration transparent? If we value community, how do we build it within institutions that control the behaviour and actions of others? How do we empower the powerless, share power and resources, and take responsibility for the outcomes? In essence, how do we transform research relationships within dominant systems when inequitable relations of power prevail? We need to attend to not only what we do, but how we do it. These are difficult questions for collaborative research teams to address. We learned that establishing a consensus on research values was a starting place in transforming research relationships, but it was not enough. As in most qualitative research, research processes must be revisited frequently. This requires continual reflection on the confirmation of active participation, commitment to research goals and processes, and commitment to ongoing collaboration and transparency. At the individual level, each team member of the research project must be reflexive of her or his own positionality and privilege within the larger research project – reflexivity is a key process that needs to engender critical reflection on our own research practices at all levels of engagement.

Although there were many challenges in this project, there were also many gifts and lessons learned. We thank all those who contributed to our learning.

REFERENCES

Fine, M., and M.E. Torre. 2004. "Re-membering Exclusions: Participatory Action Research in Public Institutions." *Qualitative Research in Psychology* 1: 15-37.

Hannah-Moffat, K. 2000. "Prisons that Empower." *British Journal of Criminology* 40: 510-31.

McTaggart, R. 1991. "Principles for Participatory Action Research." *Adult Education Quarterly* 41(3): 168-87.

Wadsworth, Yoland. 1997. *Do It Yourself Social Research*. St. Leonards, NSW: Allen and Irwin.

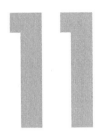

Living an Ethical Agreement
Negotiating Confidentiality and Harm in Feminist Participatory Action Research

CO L L E E N   R E I D,   PA M E L A   P O N I C,   LO U I S E
H A R A,   R O B I N   L E D R E W,   C O N N I E   K A W E E S I,
A N D   K A S H M I R   B E S L A

Developing meaningful and ethical relationships is central to community-based research and feminist methodologies (Shartrand and Brabeck 2004). Community-based and feminist approaches include the ideals of inclusion, participation, action, social change, and researcher reflexivity (Reid, Brief, and LeDrew 2009; Reid 2004). Epistemologically, this body of research is built on the assumption that important knowledge can be found in the daily lives of people in their communities and that this knowledge is always partial and context-specific (Naples 2003; Wallerstein and Duran 2003). Research informed by this perspective is conducted "with" and "for," rather than "to" or "on" people, and the development of authentic and collaborative research relationships is fundamental (Lather 1991; Tom 1997). Yet, despite the acknowledged importance of meaningful and authentic research relationships, ethical agreements often remain dictated and controlled by centralized research ethics boards (REBs) based in the academy or funding bodies. With ethical decision making held by these REBs, communities and research participants are unable to be actively involved in decisions that have a direct impact on their participation in and the actions that emerge from research. As well, this approach to navigating ethical agreements limits the ability of those of us conducting research in communities to respond to the unique, ever-changing, and context-specific needs of our projects.

In this chapter, we reflect on our experiences in conducting a two-year feminist participatory action research (FPAR) project in four diverse communities across British Columbia, Canada. We conceptualized *community* as geographical location, but understood that within the different research communities there existed communities based on identity in terms of culture, age, and relationship to the formal workforce. We discuss our experiences working between these communities elsewhere (see Reid et al. 2011). We explore how, in our efforts to protect the participants and communities from harm, we adopted a community confidentiality clause that placed serious limitations on the ability to translate the knowledge produced into meaningful actions in the communities. This tension was particularly challenging in a project specifically designed to promote local research and action.

To better understand the basis for the community confidentiality agreement that was struck in our project, we provide an overview of relevant literature in ethics and feminist participatory action research. We then discuss the evolution of the project, the project itself, and the methodological and ethical decisions that were made by the researchers and the REB. We describe the chronology of "ethical decision making" in our project that culminated in a decision reached by the REB – that we maintain community confidentiality – and then provide an analysis of how this decision created tensions in the project around issues of control, power, knowledge generation, and knowledge transfer. We conclude with some thoughts on how REBs and community and academic researchers can work together towards reaching agreements that both respect the autonomy of research communities and individuals while maintaining a research project with ethical integrity.

Feminist Participatory Action Research

Community-based research (CBR) approaches are strategies for creating knowledge that is relevant to a community's needs and interests (Gibson, Gibson, and Macaulay 2001). For decades, women's health researchers, educators, and advocates have used CBR to make space for women to speak about their oppression and their silencing, and we have offered strategies for achieving transformational actions and social change (Reid, Brief, and LeDrew 2009). Feminist participatory action research is an approach to CBR and a theory of how research can be conducted from an explicitly feminist perspective (Reid and Frisby 2008; Harding 1987; Maguire 2001). Maguire asks, "Without a grounding in feminisms, what would action research liberate us from and transform our communities into?" (2001, 60). FPAR is driven by a social justice agenda that seeks to uncover and redress inequitable power relations that manifest in the everyday lives of historically marginalized women (Lykes and Coquillon 2006). Community control over the production of knowledge is central to facilitating action towards social change. Researchers take on facilitative roles, rather than sitting back as distant observers or attempting to control the entire process. Ideally, in FPAR, participants are actively involved in all stages of knowledge production, including identifying the research problem, collecting and analyzing the data, and translating the knowledge (Frisby et al. 2005).

Conducting FPAR requires academic researchers to relinquish some of their power within the research process and to facilitate community control. While doing so more explicitly positions FPAR within a feminist social justice agenda, it also makes the work more complex because of the necessity to interrogate, redefine, and transform traditional power relations within both the research process and broader social relations. Increasingly, feminist participatory action researchers are writing about the inevitable tensions and messiness of partnering with community members for social change and interrupting established research practices and paradigms (Frisby, Maguire, and Reid 2009; Lykes, Blanche, and Hamber 2003; Maguire 1993; Ponic 2007; Reid 2004). Yet, insufficient attention has been paid to the ethical dilemmas that arise in feminist and other forms of action research, particularly in terms of how agendas of community control and social justice can be interrupted by top-down ethical review requirements.

Ethics in Feminist Participatory Action Research

Ethical considerations in research typically require researchers to ensure informed and voluntary consent, anonymity and confidentiality, and transparency (Christians 2005; Flinders 1992). Most often, ethical requirements are regulated by university and other institutional research ethics boards, which interrogate researchers' intentions and processes and seek ways of weighing the ratio of risk versus reward. It is of the utmost importance to consider the ethical parameters in research processes, so that participants are not put at undue risk, coerced, manipulated, or otherwise harmed for the sake of knowledge production. Nonetheless, the ethical decisions that researchers face are contextualized by existing and changing relationships, competing world views, and historical power dynamics. They are not straightforward equations that can be simply applied through blanket REB policies. In particular, "action research raises a unique set of ethical challenges, many of which have been overlooked in the literature" (Brydon-Miller, Greenwood, and Eikeland 2006, 129) and, from our perspective, have also been neglected by REB requirements. The deep relationships that can develop between academic researchers, community researchers, and research participants engaging in FPAR raise specific contradictions in REB rules around coercion, voluntary consent, and confidentiality, and these actually work against FPAR principles. Maintaining anonymity, for example, can compromise feminist analysis practices of contextualizing data within social, economic, and political dynamics that are, in part, provided by participants' identities and lived realities (Fine and Weis 2005; Ponic 2007). We cannot assume that all participants desire confidentiality; in fact, some prefer to have their voices heard and validated – especially if their agenda is taking action towards social change.

These ethical dilemmas and contradictions stem from the question of who controls and has power over research processes. While FPAR ideals espouse community control, most often the power in ethical decision making remains firmly held by academic researchers and institutional REBs (Lincoln 2005; Shartrand and Brabeck 2004). In large part, REBs' power is maintained because their practices and decisions are framed by traditional, positivist, and patriarchal epistemologies that assume that those in the academy are better able to "protect" participants from undue harm than the participants are able to do themselves. Eikeland (2006) refers to this as "condescending ethics," which have the effect of positioning participants as "Other," reinforcing their powerlessness, and further marginalizing them within knowledge production processes (Lincoln 2005). Such "Othering" effects are in direct conflict with FPAR ideals that espouse inclusion, participation, and liberation (Lykes and Coquillon 2006; Reid 2004). Yet, the contradictions between REB policies and FPAR principles are not clear-cut. In some situations, REBs are beginning to grapple with the unique ethical tensions associated with action research and to develop more appropriate policies, as this REB "Action Research Guidelines" example illustrates:

> One major concern in evaluating the ethics of human research is safeguarding and protecting the rights of participants in the research. This becomes particularly important in participatory, action or practitioner research when ... [d]ual relationships exist between researcher and participant, especially when people in positions of power or status undertake research in addition to their already established roles and responsibilities ... [and] information and results obtained regarding "practice" is [sic] made public through research presentations, publications, etc. (Office of Research Services 2003, 1)

Although this REB is making efforts to explicitly recognize that action research has unique ethical considerations, it remains embedded in a traditional perspective that positions academic researchers as guardians of the participants' safety and, therefore, maintains their power base. On the other hand, while top-down REB regulations can limit the potential of FPAR, Boser (2006) suggests that external rules are necessary to shed light on the often invisible power dynamics that exist in action research relationships. Given the complexity of negotiating power dynamics and ethical decisions in FPAR, researchers and participants require ways in which to think about the ethical parameters from which to balance competing needs and divergent responsibilities.

The Women's Employability and Health Project

In 2004, a group of organizations and individuals concerned about how government policy was affecting women's ability to survive financially formed the Coalition for Women's Economic Advancement. Coalition members knew that women with scarce resources had little recourse to protection through labour laws, that they were often limited to working multiple jobs paying below minimum wage, and that they were put into compromising positions that threatened their health and safety and exposed them to violence. Among the coalition organizations' members,[1] there was anecdotal evidence that provincial policy changes had resulted in an increasing number of women staying in abusive relationships; getting into sexually exploitative relationships for economic benefit; engaging in sex trade work or the underground economy; relying on their children for money, food, and shelter; and getting involved in other criminal or marginal behaviour that was directly linked to their deepening poverty. It had also been observed that the women affected were diverse ethnically, racially, socially, and geographically.

Since the coalition's formation, we acknowledged the need to better understand and document how women were coping in this deteriorating context. In this project we examined women's employability and how women's efforts to survive financially affected their health and well-being. We defined *employability* as women's relationship to the formal and informal economies, including how women "made ends meet." Inherent in our approach was a social model of women's health that recognized the social, economic, and environmental determinants of health. We aimed to examine the social context of women's health by exploring and legitimizing women's own experiences, challenging medical dominance in understandings of health, and explaining women's health in terms of their subordination and marginalization (Benoit and Shumka 2009; Morrow, Hankivsky, and Varcoe 2007; Walters 1991).

The coalition was awarded research funding to conduct feminist participation action research in the four communities for two years.[2] In choosing the research communities, the coalition considered the gap between women's and men's incomes, the sources of income in the community, and the percentage of community members dependent on transfer payments. The research communities represented British Columbia's social, economic, cultural, and geographical diversities; we characterized them as Rural-Farming, Urban–South Asian, Northern-Resource, and Remote-Reserve. In each community we hired community researchers who were trained to gather information to provide contextual information; record and transcribe the experiences of fifteen to twenty women locally by conducting one-on-one interviews and focus groups; record field notes; ensure that individual confidentiality was maintained through the use of pseudonyms and by stripping interview transcripts of any identifying information; use Atlas.ti to manage, organize, and code their data sets; and write a final research report.

The community researchers formed and worked with advisory committees (ACs) in their communities. Advisory committee members were people who worked in community organizations, municipal politics, the Chamber of Commerce, and in one town, the mayor. The ACs met three to five times over the course of the project to vet the research report that the community researchers produced. The ACs ensured that the reports did not contain information that could harm the reputation of the community or information that could identify individual women.

Over the course of the project, the community researchers communicated with each other through teleconference calls and a two-day workshop in January 2007. As principal investigator (PI), Colleen imposed an overall structure to the project – including the FPAR framework, an outline for the final community report, and training on data collection and analysis. In the beginning, Colleen envisioned the structure as more fluid and emergent; however, quickly it was apparent that the community researchers wanted structure, guidelines, and firm direction. From the outset, it was evident that the broad structure of the project and the communities involved raised a number of ethical questions. Each community had its own ethical concerns. Rural-Farming was concerned with being portrayed as the "pot-growing capital of BC," Remote-Reserve was aware of the potentially sensitive nature of the findings and the stigmatizing effect they could have on Aboriginal women, Northern-Resource knew that revelations about women's situations could be potentially explosive, and Urban–South Asian was acutely aware of negative stereotypes of the South Asian community, particularly in the wake of a number of interpartner murders. We agreed that the community researchers had to make decisions that worked for their citizens and that the ACs were in place to ensure that the communities and research participants were protected from harm. Yet, the promise of "protection" of the advisory committees was problematic. While the community researchers had been tasked with forming the ACs, and we saw their role as essential, we were also concerned that our research findings not be silenced or controlled. None of the research communities were homogeneous; within each there were inequalities and opposing perspectives and experiences. We also recognized that some interests, and not necessarily the interests of the women we hoped to hear from, may be protected under the guise of community control. We were aware of these ethical dilemmas from the beginning, and recognized that we would be unable to "solve" them all; rather, our goal was to strive continuously to engage in research with ethical integrity.

The reflections that follow are the result of an ongoing and collaborative partnership between Colleen, the lead researcher, Louise, the project coordinator, Pamela, a research consultant for the project, and some of the community researchers, including Robin, Connie, and Kashmir; see Reid et al. (2011) for an intersectional analysis of our working relationships. To this chapter, we each have contributed our own reflections, which are referenced as, for example, "Kashmir, e-mail." When a community researcher is cited who is not a co-author here, we reference her as "Researcher: Northern-Resource, field notes."

Managing an Ethical Agreement: The Fallout from the Community Confidentiality Clause

We applied for ethical review to Simon Fraser University (SFU) and to the funding foundation's research ethics board.[3] SFU approved our application within a few days. Shortly after submitting the foundation's REB forms, Colleen had a long conversation with members of that REB regarding our application. The ethical concerns that the REB raised were threefold: (1) we were asking highly sensitive questions that could result in marginalized women revealing their involvement in criminalized work, working "under the table," or defrauding the welfare system; (2) we were working in small communities where it would be difficult or impossible to ensure that women's identities would be protected by using pseudonyms and stripping data of identifying information; and (3) we were conducting research on a reserve with Aboriginal women. At that time, Colleen and the REB agreed that in order to adequately protect the participants and communities, the identities of the communities would remain confidential. When Colleen communicated this decision to the community researchers, they were un-clear about how to proceed. At that time Remote-Reserve was the only com-munity that would have chosen to keep their community confidential. We received funding to conduct FPAR, and we placed a heavy emphasis on sup-porting advocacy and actions that arose in the communities. The major form of action that was supported by the grant was the publication of com-munity research reports. The purpose of these reports was to provide evi-dence for local citizens and service providers to support their efforts to apply for funding for additional programs and future research projects. After many communications with the hired researchers about the implica-tions of this clause, in an e-mail to the funders, Colleen wrote:

> Does "not naming" the communities in documentation include all docu-ments produced by the community researchers? The challenge is that one of the intentions is for the community reports to help support local service providers, activists, and community members. For instance, we hoped that the reports could facilitate local service providers' efforts in securing more funds for relevant programs. If the community researchers are required to keep the name of the community confidential at all stages, their jobs are then more difficult because the first report's goal was to provide a context-ual overview. Do you have examples of how this has been done effectively, while still enabling and supporting local efforts? For instance, how can this be a feminist action research project, engendering participation from the community, if it is not to be communicated that the research is being done in this particular community? On what are the actions to be based, if not the outcomes of the research process and findings? Also, since no one is to know which communities have been researched, does that bar the com-munity researchers themselves from disclosing even the fact that they are undertaking this research to anyone who identifies them with their com-munity? And finally, if no community is to be identified, does this make redundant the process of obtaining Band approval for research reports, or conversely, does it extend their domain over intellectual property to the whole community, or the whole project? (Colleen, e-mail)

In response to the concerns detailed in this e-mail, Colleen organized a tele-conference with Louise, the community researchers, a representative from the foundation, and two members of the foundation's REB. At that time, we gained some clarity regarding how to conduct FPAR while maintaining community confidentiality. We agreed that the researchers would generate a research report in which the community was named. This final report could then be used *locally* to support and promote local actions. In contexts where audiences were provincial, national, or international, the communities could not be named. Yet, as the research unfolded, the community confidentiality agreement that we struck with the foundation's REB was increasingly called into question. We have discussed these tensions at length, and what follows is our analysis of them.

"Condescending Ethics": Issues of Power and Control

Conducting FPAR means deliberately confronting and attempting to re-dress dominant power relations (Reid 2004; Reid and Frisby 2008). This can be accomplished when academic researchers relinquish some aspects of control and power over the research process to local communities and re-search participants. Yet, increasingly within the ethical requirements of this project, power and control were maintained by the academic researcher and funders. As we discussed the implications of the community confidentiality clause, we wondered: *Who gets to make decisions? Who has control, and how is the community affected?* Connie characterized this decision as "southern policies" that dictated work in the north:

> My values of community empowerment were challenged, and I felt frus-trated. Always, dealing with agencies in the south [of the province], making decisions for the north [of the province]. Not understanding how the north works, how we are flexible, resourceful, and need autonomy. Northern people have a pride in making their own way, taking control of their deci-sions, and working cooperatively with each other. Dependence on set poli-cies from external agents is difficult. In future, I will definitely ask more questions and have a clear understanding of the expectations of the project. (Connie, field notes)

Not only did Connie feel that the REB was imposing a heavy-handed man-date on them, but she also felt that such a decision would limit the capacity that could be built in smaller and more remote communities if decision making was held afar by a research ethics board.

Foremost in my mind is the need to train local northern researchers to build community capacity for further research. This project did tie into my past experience, and I really felt that a community researcher should conduct the work; call it northern pride, if you want. I always have a great deal of northern pride and loyalty. There was a real community commitment to the project, and I think this will help the community-based community researchers. It also works well with the participatory research method, and I always enjoy working collaboratively with groups and individuals. (Connie, field notes)

Although all of the researchers understood the very real risks that women in their communities faced in their participation in the project, Connie and Robin reflected that the ethical review process felt tedious and that it was not meaningful to their local contexts and goals:

We were constantly negotiating and revisiting the ethical restraints of confidentiality that confront FPAR. The negotiations between the funders, the university, the head researchers, and the local research team were still underway long after our first, broadly advertised public meeting. (Robin, field notes)

Once we start the project, we can have a better answer to the questions, especially around collective vs. individual confidentially. I have been reading the e-mails, from Colleen to the foundation, and still feel a sense of external or systemic control over the project. I understand the need for consistency and a clear policy on confidentiality, but I do not agree with the statements of the REB. Perhaps, it is not my place to agree or disagree; maybe I am taking too much ownership for the project at this stage. Perhaps I should start to think of ways to relinquish my role in the project ... FPAR is built on the assumption that the grassroots community is actively involved in all stages of the research project. The definition of the "community" should be the local community, because it is here that the research action must be implemented. Small, rural, and remote northern communities require the community capacity to be autonomous and to integrate shared norms around issues of community ownership and confidentiality. (Connie, field notes)

Importantly, Connie questioned if it was "her place" to agree or disagree with the REB's decision. She felt disempowered in the ethics review process by the control wielded by the REB and by Colleen, as the project's principal investigator.

From a different perspective, Kashmir felt the community confidentiality clause would be difficult to explain and rationalize to participants and would, consequently, make it difficult to recruit them:

> Balancing the importance of individual confidentiality and creating opportunities for action and advocacy in FPAR can be a challenging experience. The funders for the Women's Employability and Health Project required that the communities in which the research took place be kept confidential in the outcome reports. By following this requirement, important contextual information and analysis would be compromised. South Asian women living in [name of city] were one of the groups that were interviewed for this project. Asking a minority group that is not familiar with ideas of research and evaluation to take part in such a project presented many challenges. Women needed to feel safe in sharing their ideas and experiences. If they had ideas for needs and change, and were told that they as a group would not be identified because of confidentiality reasons, why would they want to participate? (Kashmir, field notes)

The ethics review process was unfamiliar to participants in the South Asian community, and being forced to engage in prolonged conversations about ethics was potentially a deterrent for South Asian women's involvement in the project. When Kashmir asked, "if they had ideas for needs and change, and were told that they as a group would not be identified," she also suggests that this practice would silence South Asian women's experiences and perpetuate their invisibility in the research literature.

It is also possible to view the REB's mandate as an imperialist and paternalistic "handing down," or what Eikeland (2006) coined as "condescending" ethics, that did not take into account cultural norms or gender dynamics within local communities. Both SFU's and the foundation's REBs required that we receive approval from the Band Council. In our particular case, seeking Band approval did little to protect the individual women involved in the research. At the time of our application to Band Council, all of the band members were men. The community researcher speculated that we might have difficulty gaining project approval because the research could potentially reveal violence and drug and alcohol abuse in the community:

Once they were convinced that we would be respectful and meant to give women local control of how the research would be done, local women were very excited at the prospect of gaining a meaningful picture of what it means to live and work in their community. Very little research of this nature exists, and they have rarely had the use of the findings from all the previous research done on their community. They hoped this would make a big difference for them in understanding women's experiences better, advocating for meaningful responses, and accessing resources from all sources. The contradiction in where permission to do research on traditional lands is sought put a wrench into this, and that was exacerbated by the community confidentiality requirement. First Nations tradition places women in an esteemed position, but the ethics guidelines require permission from local Band governors, who are all men. Permission was granted by the Band Council to do research, as long as individual women's and the community's confidentiality is preserved. Some local women shared with us that by bypassing the matriarchs and by ensuring community confidentiality, men in the community could continue to control with impunity what was learned of how they behave locally and how that knowledge is shared. We also heard undocumented stories of how some women were sexually assaulted and harassed in local Band offices. The coalition did not seek to ensure that the Matriarchs' permission was sought, but we supported the notion of having two Matriarchs (Elders) participate on the advisory committee. (Researcher: Remote-Reserve, field notes)

By placing the ethical process in the hands of a male-dominated Band Council, women's ability to control the research locally was compromised and undermined.

In all of these cases, we acknowledged that the REB's decision was well intentioned and aimed to protect the women who participated in the research. However, for gender, cultural, and geographical reasons, the blanket policy applied by the REB effectively maintained power over the community researchers and how they engaged with their research participants. It placed Colleen in a position of communicating and interpreting the REB's decision for the local communities, while bearing responsibility for ensuring that those working on the project locally understood and respected the ethical parameters of their work and the potentially negative consequences of breaching ethical decisions. Finally, the imposition of community confidentiality from an REB on community researchers, when it is neither the community researchers' desire nor choice, suggests that those in the community who have been working intimately with the project are not in a position to understand research ethics or to decide what is best for their community.

Constraints on Knowledge Generation and Knowledge Translation

Central to feminist participatory action research is the commitment to using the knowledge created through the research process to take action that is relevant and meaningful to local communities (Reid and Frisby 2008). As each researcher gathered data, engaged in data analysis, and began to think about report writing, dissemination, and initiating local actions, she began to question: *If research is about knowledge generation and knowledge transfer, is it desirable to restrict the circulation of findings from a research report? Is it possible to engage in local actions and activism if one is required to maintain community confidentiality?* Kashmir had been inspired to do research because she had struggled with finding information about South Asian women's experiences in her community. She felt that the most important action to emerge from this project would be the research report itself:

> By asking that the ethnicity and community demographics be kept out of the outcomes, this would take away from the many needs which may have been identified. Given that so little research is conducted in regards to issues faced by this cultural group, why would it be beneficial to keep that useful information unidentified? (Kashmir, field notes)

Similarly, Connie was inspired to take on this project because of the feminist values it espoused:

> In the beginning I took on this project to hear the voices of women. To make some change for women in my community. Most of the women we interviewed did not want to use a pseudonym and wanted their voices heard by other women. I think this experience has led me to understand the meaning of the breadth and richness of the women's experiences and reminds me that all women have meaning to their stories. In this fast-paced world, we often do not have the time or energy to reflect on the meaning of experiences, words, and symbolic meaning to our thoughts. (Connie, e-mail)

Connie felt that the research would only be meaningful if it remained embedded in its local context. And, certainly, many feminist and action researchers have recognized that applying a social and contextual analysis to local findings is the researcher's key job in uncovering patterns of systemic marginalization and inequity (Fine and Weis 2005; Tom and Herbert 2001). So little was (and is) known about northern Canadian women's experiences in a resource town that to remove the local context would dilute the findings:

> From my own professional background of social work, maintaining individual confidentiality is very clear and guided by the British Columbia Social Work Code of Ethics. I think that from the onset of the project there was a lack of clarity on the issue of confidentially. I was very surprised that the community researchers could not mention the names of the communities involved in the project. In particular, I did not understand the rationale from [funders] for not contextualizing the research communities. (Connie, e-mail)

From the beginning, the Rural-Farming community had a large and strong contingent of community women interested in taking action. As local actions emerged over the course of Rural-Farming's project, the community researchers were confused about what they could do and say:

> The issue of transportation barriers emerged in our first meeting and was documented in our first report. Two nursing students, hearing of our project, approached us in September 2006 to do an associated piece of research and action for a course at [name of university]. Our local research team suggested they explore the transportation issue in more detail. With less than sixty-five days available, the nursing students did an impressive survey of local transportation needs. Since part of their mandate was to include the lobbying process, they presented their report to local and regional politicians and newspapers. Their work resulted in a small but significant change to the local transit system, which expanded its schedule. This action proceeded in spite of an e-mail discussion between the funders of the research project and the head researcher, who attempted to control (perhaps "protect" is a better word) community confidentiality ... This concern about community confidentiality prevented our project from being associated with this successful piece of action. Two years have passed since the enthusiastic public presentation of the research project in our town. Although other pieces of action, both individual and group, have resulted from our activities, we have not been able to take much, if any, credit for

them. The unfortunate consequence has been to limit the credibility of the research project as a vehicle for action among interested women and our advisory committee. We have yet to see whether this cynicism can be counteracted following the release of the final report. (Robin, field notes)

The ongoing deliberations between the funders, Colleen, and the researchers in the Rural-Farming community on generating local actions and maintaining community confidentiality had the unfortunate effect of raising doubts about the credibility of the project locally. If the FPAR project could not pursue local actions unencumbered, what was the use of the project in the first place? Why would women locally have invested their energy and hopes into the project only for it to remain hamstrung by what was perceived as academic ethical debates?

As Colleen heard of these frustrations, it became increasingly obvious that the community confidentiality clause placed significant limitations on what could be said about or what could emerge from the research. Within a year of initiating the project, the community researchers, Colleen, Pamela, and Louise began co-presenting at local, provincial, and national conferences. We also began co-writing. At a provincial gathering with women's health researchers, Colleen and Connie co-presented the findings from the Northern-Resource community. After our presentation, one of the participants expressed interest in reading the report from the Remote-Reserve community because she felt that the questions we asked were important and relevant to her own First Nations community. With the community confidentiality clause in mind, Colleen declined this opportunity for sharing the findings. Given that Remote-Reserve was producing this community report, Colleen wondered: *Would the hired researcher from Remote-Reserve be able to send her community report to someone in a different community? How can this be controlled?*

While this kind of knowledge sharing and capacity building can be viewed as a successful outcome of any feminist participatory action research project, the community confidentiality clause put a "gag order" on the community researchers' active dissemination of research findings. In public forums such as conferences and workshops, attendees know the identities of the presenters. Therefore, the identity of the communities cannot remain confidential. The community researchers expressed an ongoing interest in co-authoring manuscripts for academic journals and book chapters, co-presenting at workshops and conferences, and remaining engaged with efforts to disseminate the findings. In the spirit of FPAR, the sustained involvement of community researchers, all of whom continue to be excited by their involvement in the research, should be supported and encouraged. FPAR aims to ensure that knowledge contributes to making a positive change in the world. If opportunities for sharing findings are lost because of a community confidentiality clause, then the impact of the research is limited substantially.

Academic Control of Ethical Decision Making

Shortly before Colleen and Connie were due to co-present, Connie, who is a strong advocate for women's health in her community, told Colleen that she was writing a letter to the foundation indicating her intention to name her community in the conference presentation. She wrote:

> I have decided to disclose the name of the community ... many of the women expressed an interest in other communities hearing their stories ... The Community Advisory Committee is supportive of sharing the research findings and recommendations with other northern communities. There is a need for northern women to understand and listen to research conducted in northern communities. In addition, without the context of the community the recommendations could not be understood in a northern and remote community. I appreciate your understanding of the significance and importance for northern communities to conduct research that will be applicable to other northern communities. (Connie, e-mail)

Colleen was contacted immediately by the program manager of the foundation. What ensued were a number of telephone conversations and e-mails about Connie "contravening" the ethical agreement that was reached nine months prior. The program manager, in consultation with the foundation's chair of the REB, agreed that Colleen could write an amendment letter to the REB. Within days, Colleen received a letter stating:

> The ... Research Ethics Board has reviewed your request for an amendment to the ethics certificate and approved the requested change: that community researchers, with the support and agreement of their Advisory Committees, will be able to name their communities, in any context they choose, with the exception of academic journal articles.

The clause "with the exception of academic journal articles" maintained relations of inequality by enforcing confidentiality when the work was shared in academic publications outside the community. Indeed, the community researchers did not have full control over the findings from the research in their communities. Regardless, as a research team, we felt vindicated: for the most part, we were now able to make decisions that were appropriate for the research communities and that enabled us to freely continue our knowledge translation activities. It is noteworthy that the foundation's REB was only willing to engage with the principal investigator (Colleen) about these issues. Although Connie wrote the initial letter that inspired the amendment, she was effectively removed from the conversation and made invisible in the process. Colleen, as the academic (read: legitimate) researcher, was positioned as the gatekeeper to ethical decision making.

Implications: Towards Living an Ethical Agreement

Our intention in writing this chapter was not to portray all research ethics boards as unnecessarily and uncompromisingly wielding control over communities who are engaged in research. Nor are we suggesting that communities are always capable of negotiating the thorny ethical issues that can arise in conducting feminist participatory action research in one's own community. We recognize that there are always going to be challenges in achieving our lofty FPAR goals of participation, inclusivity, and shared decision making. As well, we have always understood the fundamental concerns that led the foundation's REB to ask that we maintain community confidentiality: this decision was based on a genuine concern for the safety of the local research participants and the possible stigmatization of the communities. However, ethical requirements are always political, as they are always infused with power (Hilsen 2006). Do those who control ethical agreements also bear the responsibility for maintaining them? What happens, or what is lost, when the imposition of a "condescending ethics" framework results in ethical decisions being handed down? In the context of FPAR's goals of capacity building, partnering meaningfully with people in the community, and informing action and social change, the imposition of community confidentiality imposed major limitations on our research project.

Through our ongoing efforts to understand the risks faced by our research participants, and the measures necessary to protect them, we gained a deeper and more sophisticated understanding of the ethical considerations involved in any FPAR project. FPAR processes demand an unsettling of traditional relationships in research. No longer does the researcher maintain control over the research under the presumption of "objectivity," and no longer are participants passively involved as "subjects." It follows that no longer are REBs able to maintain control over how decisions are made and implemented in the local research communities. What is required is a fundamental shift in how REBs relate to these experiential forms of research that aim to transgress all layers and forms of power and control.

The main purpose of considering ethics in any kind of research is to provide safety for participants and to minimize their risk. While this is of paramount importance, in the context of a FPAR project, who gets to define what is safe? How are measures of safety applied across diverse communities and participants? What happens if participants or communities are willing to accept some degree of risk in order to be involved in the research and to create change? Certainly, in some instances, participants may prefer to have their voices heard and validated (Giordano et al. 2007; Reid 2004). As well, feminists have challenged masculinist approaches to ethics for their minimalist notions of "do no harm" to include a discussion of "do some good" with the research. In order to confront the hegemonies of gender, race, and class relations, feminists have long argued that researchers have a responsibility to contribute to social justice – a reframing that Lather (1991) refers to as "catalytic validity." If FPAR is about creating new knowledge paradigms and transferring power from researcher to participants, from academia to the community, then these shifts must also flow through the ethical agreements that are reached. Decisions around community and individual confidentiality must be co-created, contextualized, and transparent. Researchers and research ethics boards must trust that participants know their own boundaries and that they can be responsible for creating dialogues that explore the costs and benefits of their involvement in the research. Just as FPAR advocates partnerships and sharing power, it is possible to strike this kind of balance in the ethical decision-making process. Funding bodies, research ethics boards, academic researchers, community researchers, and research participants must share both the control and responsibility for research ethics. This requires constant communication, and although it can make the process laborious, this communication can result in richer and more meaningful research relationships for all who are willing and able to engage in them.

We titled this chapter "Living an Ethical Agreement" because it reflects what we learned in our work: in any FPAR project, research ethics and the power dynamics that contextualize them must be taken seriously, discussed frequently, and become an integral part of each stage of the research. Ethical frameworks must be manifested in every micro-decision that is made throughout the research process (Brydon-Miller, Greenwood, and Eikeland 2006). *Living an ethical agreement* requires that research ethics boards, academic researchers, and researchers working in their communities engage with each other to understand how ethical issues arise and unfold in local contexts. Eikeland (2006) refers to this as "communities of practice," such that all involved participate in conversations and decisions about ethical parameters. It demands constant attention and vigilance, and the development of a respectful and sustained partnership between REBs and those who require their approval, to conduct important and meaningful work.

Fundamentally, ethics is about the rules of behaviour and human duty, morals and values, understanding right and wrong, justice and injustice, good and bad, and doing the right thing (Australian Government 2005). REBs, academic and community researchers, and participants all have a role to play in this conversation. They share a mutual responsibility for "living an ethical agreement," for engaging continuously in understanding how research decisions are made and how power relations are negotiated towards the best interests and goals of participants and communities.

NOTES

1 The organizations that were involved in the coalition were local social service agencies with explicit mandates for serving and supporting women.
2 We received a seed grant for Colleen and Louise to travel to the research communities to discuss the proposed project to solicit input. From these visits we learned that the questions we posed were meaningful and important to people locally. Once we secured the full research grant, we hired researchers in the research communities. Colleen and Louise worked closely with the community researchers. They provided research training, guidance, support, and resources, as well as assistance with the research budgets and other kinds of logistical support.
3 Simon Fraser University was the institution where Colleen was doing her postdoctoral fellowship at that time.

REFERENCES

Australian Government. 2005. *Keeping Research on Track: A Guide for Aboriginal and Torres Strait People about Health and Research Ethics*. Canberra: National Health and Medical Research Council and the Australian Health Ethics Committee. http://www.nhmrc.gov.au.

Benoit, Cecilia, and Leah Shumka. 2009. *Gendering the Health Determinants Framework: Why Girls' and Women's Health Matters*. Vancouver: Women's Health Research Network.

Boser, Susan. 2006. "Ethics and Power in Community-Campus Partnerships for Research." *Action Research* 4(1): 9-21.

Brydon-Miller, Mary, David Greenwood, and Olav Eikeland. 2006. "Strategies for Addressing Ethical Issues in Action Research." *Action Research* 4(1): 129-31.

Christians, Clifford G. 2005. "Ethics and the Politics in Qualitative Research." In N.K. Denzin and Y.S. Lincoln, eds., *Handbook of Qualitative Research*, 139-64. Thousand Oaks, CA: Sage Publications.

Eikeland, Olav. 2006. "Condescending Ethics and Action Research." *Action Research* 4(1): 37-47.

Fine, Michelle, and Lois Weis. 2005. Introduction. In M. Fine and L. Weis, eds., *Beyond Silenced Voices: Class, Race and Gender in United States Schools*, xi-xiv. New York: State University of New York Press.

Flinders, David J. 1992. "In Search of Ethical Guidance: Constructing a Basis for Dialogue." *Qualitative Studies in Education* 5(2): 101-15.

Frisby, Wendy, Patricia Maguire, and Colleen Reid. 2009. "The 'F' Word Has Everything to Do with It: How Feminist Theories Inform Action Research." *Action Research* 7(1): 13-29.

Frisby, Wendy, Colleen Reid, Sydney Millar, and Larena Hoeber. 2005. "Putting 'Participatory' into Participatory Forms of Action Research." *Journal of Sport Management* 19(1): 367-96.

Gibson, Nancy, G. Gibson, and Ann Macaulay. 2001. "Community-Based Research: Negotiating Agendas and Evaluating Outcomes." In J. Morse, J. Swanson, and A.J. Kuzel, eds., *The Nature of Qualitative Evidence*, 160-82. Thousand Oaks, CA: Sage Publications.

Giordano, James, Michelle O'Reilly, Helen Taylor, and Nisha Dogra. 2007. "Confidentiality and Autonomy: The Challenge(s) of Offering Research Participants a Choice of Disclosing Their Identity." *Qualitative Health Research* 17(2): 264-75.

Harding, Sandra. 1987. "Is There a Feminist Method?" In S. Harding, ed., *Feminism and Methodology*, 1-14. Bloomington, IN: Open University Press.

Hilsen, Anne Inga. 2006. "And They Shall Be Known by Their Deeds: Ethics and Politics in Action Research." *Action Research* 4(1): 23-36.

Lather, Patti. 1991. *Getting Smart: Feminist Research and Pedagogy within the Postmodern*. New York: Routledge, Chapman and Hall.

Lincoln, Yvonna S. 2005. "Institutional Review Boards and Methodological Conservatism." In N.K. Denzin and Y.S. Lincoln, eds., *Handbook of Qualitative Research*, 165-81. Thousand Oaks, CA: Sage Publications.

Lykes, M. Brinton, Martin Terre Blanche, and Brandon Hamber. 2003. "Narrating Survival and Change in Guatemala and South Africa: The Politics of Representation and a Liberatory Community Psychology." *American Journal of Community Psychology* 31(1-2): 79-90.

Lykes, M. Brinton, and Erzulie Coquillon. 2001. "Uneven Ground: Feminisms and Action Research." In P. Reason and H. Bradbury, eds., *Handbook of Action Research: Participative Inquiry and Practice*, 59-69. London: Sage Publications.

–. 2006. "Participatory and Action Research and Feminisms: Towards Transformative Praxis." In S. Hesse-Biber, ed., *Handbook of Feminist Research: Theory and Praxis*, 297-326. Thousand Oaks, CA: Sage Publications.

Morrow, Marina, Olena Hankivsky, and Colleen Varcoe, eds. 2007. *Women's Health in Canada: Critical Perspectives on Theory and Policy.* Toronto: University of Toronto Press.

Naples, Nancy. 2003. *Feminism and Method: Ethnography, Discourse Analysis and Activist Research.* New York: Routledge.

Office of Research Services. 2003. *Behavioural Research Ethics Board Forms and Guidance Notes: Appendix 3: Action Research Guidelines.* Vancouver, BC, University of British Columbia. http://www.ors.ubc.ca/ethics/forms/BREBpercent 20Appendixpercent203percent20(Actionpercent20Research).doc.

Ponic, Pamela. 2007. "Embracing Complexity in Community-Based Health Promotion: Inclusion, Power and Women's Health." PhD diss., University of British Columbia, Vancouver, BC.

Reid, Colleen. 2004. *The Wounds of Exclusion: Poverty, Women's Health, and Social Justice.* Walnut Creek, CA: Left Coast Press.

Reid, Colleen, Elana Brief, and Robin LeDrew. 2009. *Our Common Ground: Cultivating Women's Health through Community-Based Research.* Vancouver, BC: Women's Health Research Network.

Reid, Colleen, and Wendy Frisby. 2008. "Continuing the Journey: Articulating Dimensions of Feminist Participatory Action Research." In P. Reason and H. Bradbury, eds., *Handbook of Action Research,* 2nd ed., 93-105. London: Sage Publications.

Reid, Colleen, Pamela Ponic, Louise Hara, Connie Kaweesi, and Robin LeDrew. 2011. "Performing Intersectionality: The Mutuality of Intersectional Analysis and Feminist Participatory Action Health Research." In O. Hankivsky, ed., *Health Inequities in Canada: Intersectional Frameworks and Practices,* 92-111. Vancouver, BC: UBC Press.

Shartrand, Angela, and Mary M. Brabeck. 2004. "An Examination of Collaborative Research in Light of the APA Code of Ethics and Feminist Ethics." In M. Brydon-Miller, P. Maguire, and A. McIntyre, eds., *Traveling Companions: Feminism, Teaching, and Action Research,* 137-56. Westport, CT: Praeger.

Tom, Allison. 1997. "The Deliberate Relationship: A Frame for Talking about Faculty-Student Relationships." *Alberta Journal of Educational Research* 43(1): 3-21.

Tom, Allison, and Carol Herbert. 2001. "The Near Miss: A Story of Relationship." *Qualitative Inquiry* 8(3): 591-607.

Wallerstein, N., and B. Duran. 2003. "The Conceptual, Historical and Practical Roots of Community-Based Participatory Research and Related Participatory Traditions." In M. Minkler and N. Wallerstein, eds., *Community-Based Participatory Research for Health,* 27-52. San Francisco: Jossey-Bass.

Walters, Vivienne. 1991. "Beyond Medical and Academic Agendas: Lay Perspectives and Priorities." *Atlantis* 17(1): 28-35.

12

Capacity Building Is a Two-Way Street
Learning from Doing Research within
Aboriginal Communities

COLLEEN VARCOE, HELEN BROWN,
BETTY CALAM, MARLA J. BUCHANAN,
AND VERA NEWMAN

Calls for capacity building in research abound. In health research, the idea of capacity building is used mostly in reference to non-academic researchers, including representatives of communities or groups who are the "subjects" of research. For example, in 2004, the Canadian Institutes of Health Research (CIHR) called for HIV/AIDS Community-Based Research Program proposals with the intention to provide "the opportunity for community organizations to enhance their research skills through workshops facilitated by experienced community-based representatives and researchers" (CIHR 2004). This is an important trend; enhancing the research skills of community members and organizations can provide vital opportunities to engage communities. However, enacting capacity building as "code" for the development of non-academics involved in research implies that capacity is deficient and/or non-existent in non-academics and that capacity is built in one direction – that is, from those assumed to be more expert in research to those who are not. Framing capacity building in this way also signifies that certain forms of knowledge ought to trump other forms for research to be legitimate and rigorous.

Capacity building in this sense has become entrenched in relation to research with Aboriginal people in Canada. For example, the goal of the 2007 CIHR Guidelines for Health Research Involving Aboriginal People was "to assist researchers and institutions in carrying out ethical and culturally competent research involving Aboriginal people. The intent is to promote health through research that is in keeping with Aboriginal values and traditions." Article 2.10 of the guidelines, titled "Empowerment and Research Capacity Development," states:

> A researcher should support education and training of Aboriginal people in the community, including training in research methods and ethics. To the degree reasonably possible, a researcher should work to foster education and training of community members to enhance their participation in the research project. Researchers should, where possible, employ community members.

Again, capacity building is important and much needed. However, the underlying assumptions emphasize the importance of academic researchers as "agents" and Aboriginal people as the "targets" of capacity building. Underlying assumptions also may suggest that such efforts are inherently "good" for Aboriginal people, with little attention paid to how such strategies constitute another form of colonization. A "one way" direction is reflective of what is taken to be legitimate knowledge in research. Conventional research methodologies and protocols for research ethics are seen to be more important, for example, than knowledge and practices of local traditions, connections, and ways of living and being. Yet, the latter are rich sources of both methodological and ethical wisdom in research.

Research capacity building is related both to expanding and improving knowledge development and to ethical research. In a review of the ethical aspects of action research, Eikeland (2006) argues that conventional research ethics are insufficient for grappling with the relations between researchers and researched as enacted within action research, since it is constituted within the relations assumed by conventional research. Eikeland claims that conventional research ethics is a "condescending ethics," unfit for action research because of its practice of "Othering" human beings as research subjects. Similarly, without critical attention to underlying presuppositions conveyed by research conventions, even research that purports to be decolonizing in intent can reinscribe rather than resist and replace colonizing practices. As Tenfingers notes, "the history and legacy of Western, colonial research methodologies and policy frameworks continue to create and maintain dichotomies of superior/inferior, and valued/not valued between Western and First Nations cultures, peoples and knowledge" (2000, S60). Actions by Aboriginal communities and scholars increasingly pressure research funding organizations to recognize the colonizing history and potential of research. For example, the CIHR, the Natural Sciences and Engineering Research Council (NSERC), and the Social Sciences and Humanities Research Council (SSHRC) draft second edition of the Tri-Council Policy Statement on ethical conduct for research involving humans (Interagency Advisory Panel on Research Ethics 2008) shows some progress with respect to critiques such as those raised by Brown (2005). The policy mentions the "colonial past" and recognizes that "intrusive or insensitive research can contribute to negative stereotypes of Aboriginal peoples." However, in view of such minor gains, questions remain as to whether and how decolonizing methodologies can be enacted within Western research frameworks.

Conceptualizing and enacting capacity building as a one-way street can entrench the divide between academic researchers and Aboriginal communities, leaving unquestioned assumptions regarding the presumed superiority of academic (generally Eurocentric) knowledge and research practices and processes. Sustaining dichotomies of superior/inferior and valued/not valued is, in part, the product of presuming that Aboriginal peoples' capacities in research need "enhancing" in the first place. A decolonizing intention requires critique of all power relations, knowledge claims, and Western methodological conventions, including critique of the ways in which they reinforce the colonizing potential of research.

Academic researchers and community researchers need to assume the roles of learners and leaders at different times, for different reasons in a negotiated, dynamic process. Further, we argue that guidelines such as those produced by CIHR should go much further to account for the historical context of research with Aboriginal communities and contemporary forces that continue to create possibilities for paternalistic and exploitative practices. "Partnership" research with Aboriginal people should work towards Aboriginal leadership, management and control of research, and carefully negotiated research practices that enact respect for capacities that exist within Aboriginal communities and people. Yet, the meaning of leadership, management, and control can be interpreted differently within particular communities and are shaped by local politics. For example, the 'Namgis visiting research agreement indicates that the Band controls knowledge developed from research; however, the question of who leads the research is less clear. In our work together, leadership was continually negotiated against a backdrop of understanding that our research practices could either undermine or enhance the relevance of our findings in *both* academic and community contexts. We argue that fostering a more socially just and equitable world and creating "good" science and rigorous inquiry through partnership research requires continual negotiation of relations and practices.

Relationships, the core of research partnerships, are embedded in historical, social, and material circumstances. Thus, we argue, relationships must be developed with intention, authenticity, and transparency, with attention to power dynamics, how power dynamics are shaped by wider circumstances, and the potential for harm. Our experiences provided a unique opportunity to consider research leadership and relationships within the complex gendered, raced, and classed context of the colonial politics of Canadian society and of the communities and university associated with our study.

We write this chapter from our perspectives as five variously positioned researchers: one community researcher (Vera) and four academic researchers from different disciplines (Colleen, Helen, Betty, and Marla). We draw upon our experience working together in four First Nations communities on the Rural Aboriginal Maternity Project (RAMP). We propose that research practices need to be infused with the understanding that capacity building is a "two-way street." Although we use different languages to speak about what we have learned, together we argue that even well-intentioned capacity-building efforts can and do reinforce paternalistic and colonizing relationships with Aboriginal people. For example, when reading a draft of this chapter, Vera responded first, by saying, "You might want to start by telling me what this all means." While we share the same message, using "academic speak" to describe our project can undermine our intention to value all team members' knowledge and research skills. While Aboriginal people should benefit as much as possible from any research in which they are involved (including economically, such as through employment), and while enhancing participation is critical, academic researchers (especially non-Aboriginal academic researchers) should position themselves simultaneously as leaders and learners in relation to Aboriginal communities and peoples. Being both leaders and learners meant that, as a team of researchers, we listened for how academic research practices can, as Vera states, "make you feel like if you aren't educated in the university, your contribution is not as important." The skills, knowledge, and contributions of Aboriginal people and communities should not be overshadowed by emphasis on Eurocentric research conventions.

In this chapter, we first examine the Eurocentric, colonial, and patriarchal context of research with Aboriginal people; we then analyze what we learned about capacity building during our RAMP experiences; finally, we describe implications of our analysis for academic and community-based researchers and funding bodies, for fostering more effective capacity building. We propose rethinking capacity building as a complex relational endeavour, in which all involved seek to understand and learn from multiple perspectives, and to respect the wisdom of others. Rather than providing recipes for who should participate in research, who should lead and how, our experience suggests some guiding principles and questions that can reframe the idea of capacity – a contextual, dynamic, negotiated process that optimizes the conditions for Aboriginal leadership.

Eurocentric Research and Aboriginal People

Calls for the democratization and decolonization of research are particularly critical in relation to Aboriginal people. Historically, researchers have participated in the processes of colonizing indigenous people globally, including Aboriginal people in Canada. In the early days of colonization, European ethnographers documented the lives of Aboriginal people throughout what is now known as British Columbia, often portraying people in ways that aligned with colonizing objectives. Portraying Aboriginal people as nomadic, savage, and in need of civilizing aligned with the objectives of appropriating land and resources and cultural and religious assimilation and conversion. As Smith (1974) points out, in his introduction to *The Adventures and Sufferings of John R. Jewitt, Captive among the Nootka, 1803-1805*, such research accounts were probably very important in shaping non-Aboriginal people's opinions of Aboriginal people in North America.

Contemporary research practices often perpetuate and continue the colonizing gaze. Mechanisms to interrupt these processes, while well intentioned, often are rooted in Eurocentric paradigms, relying on academic structures such as human ethics review boards, research funding bodies, and policy instruments administered by universities. Thus, these mechanisms fall short of decolonization. For example, the Tri-Council Policy Statement on Aboriginal research ethics regarding approval mechanisms is important, but it does not address how researchers are to be held accountable at the local level, such as in Aboriginal communities. Typically, university ethics reviews involve an initial review prior to the start-up of research, and while changes are supposed to be reviewed, the onus for doing so is on academic researchers. There is no monitoring of adherence to ethical commitments articulated in ethics applications, and more importantly, the criteria for guiding and evaluating ethics are derived from conventional research (Eikeland 2006). Over the past few decades, Aboriginal academics, communities, and leaders have lobbied vigorously for self-determination in research – and the advent of research "protocols" and agreements between academics and Aboriginal communities have been important steps in attempting to prevent further exploitation and improprieties.

Globally, and in Canada, indigenous scholars and leaders have fought continuously against colonizing practices within research. Recent decades have seen significant work. For example, in 1999 Maori scholar Linda Tuhiwai Smith published her now classic book, *Decolonizing Methodologies: Research and Indigenous People,* which offered a decolonizing framework and set research with indigenous peoples within wider historical, political, and cultural contexts. In Canada, the principles of ownership, control, access, and possession (OCAP) were developed and published by the First Nations Centre to "enable self-determination over all research concerning First Nations" (First Nations Centre 2007, 1). Numerous First Nations have developed their own protocols based on these and similar principles. These works have resulted in greater awareness and interest in the colonizing potential of research and efforts to mitigate this potential. Some of this well-intentioned direction has become manifest in an emphasis on capacity building. However, the development of guidelines and agreements, and an emphasis on capacity building, may inadvertently have stunted efforts to interrogate continuously what constitutes ethical research involving Aboriginal communities and to generate what Eikeland (2006) refers to as "indigenous" criteria – that is, criteria arising from the people being studied. Further, such efforts generally have been based on dominant assumptions regarding what constitutes community, and who speaks for any given community, at times eclipsing the diverse histories and politics of particular communities that shape research processes.

Aboriginal Communities as Gendered Colonial Constructions

The question of who represents the community is one of the key challenges to any community-based research. However, this question has particular salience in relation to Aboriginal communities in Canada – communities that have been shaped by the colonizing policies emanating from the Indian Act, with particular consequences for Aboriginal women. The Indian Act, and its subsequent policies and practices, were fraught with gendered discrimination. For example, women (and their children) were disenfranchised if they married non-Aboriginal men; leadership was dictated using Eurocentric, patriarchal models that in many cases undermined women's traditional leadership roles. Subsequent policies intended to correct some of the most overtly problematic aspects of federal policy, in fact, further disenfranchised women (Fiske 1995, 2000, 2006; Fiske and Browne 2004). Consequently, gender politics in Aboriginal communities have been shaped by colonial policies, so that in some contexts women may be marginalized both within Canadian society and within Band and community politics.

The experiences of colonization and the effects of those experiences vary across the diversity of Aboriginal Nations and communities. In Canada, *Aboriginal* encompasses First Nations, Métis, and Inuit people, with more than fifty Aboriginal languages currently spoken across the country (Cook and Howe 2004). Aboriginal communities are highly diverse, and within any given community, there is a diversity of families, clans, and leadership. The meaning of community, or similarity between communities, cannot be assumed. Neither can it be assumed that "traditional" communities are static. Our project was situated within these colonial and neo-colonial dynamics, and it offered an opportunity for considering what it might mean to work in a decolonizing way together.

The Rural Aboriginal Maternity Project

The RAMP began as a relatively conventional social science research project, funded by the Canadian Institutes of Health Research, with the goal of including Aboriginal women's perspectives in research on rural maternity care. The original plans called for women in Aboriginal communities to collect data on rural Aboriginal women's maternity care experiences in the form of semi-structured interviews. The study was initiated by a team of academic researchers in partnership with four rural Aboriginal communities in British Columbia. However, part way through the study, personal, relational, and ethical issues necessitated a change in the leadership and composition of the academic team. All staff and academic researchers but two were replaced, while the configuration of the community team members remained relatively stable. Following the major shift in the academic team, one community team member left the team for personal reasons, and a woman who had been interviewed as a participant by the initial team joined the research team as a community researcher.

The triggering events that led to the change in the academic team were initially not shared with community team members. However, these circumstances contributed to a highly charged debate at the university level regarding who should lead the project forward and to what degree the personal conduct of some of the university team members signalled their trustworthiness and ethics in the wider relational research endeavour with Aboriginal communities. These circumstances had at least two key effects on the project. First, Vera explains:

> It became next to impossible to believe that the research would be conducted in a respectful way after a seven-month period of no communication with no response to our calls from the original team. We were "sold" on how great the research would be for our community, and then we heard nothing for months. This made me question if the team would really be respectful of the participants. Unless people are treated well, I could not feel good about recruiting those mothers into the study. They didn't need disrespectful treatment on top of everything else.

Second, the reformulated team brought different theoretical perspectives into the foreground of the project. While the academic team change necessitated building new relationships, and attempting to repair damage done to trust by the antecedent events, the changes also provided opportunities. The project shifted from a relatively conventional study to a more action-oriented and participatory project with an explicit anti-colonial stance, informed by previous experience working in partnership with Aboriginal communities, and by critical feminist, post-colonial, and indigenous thinking. For example, the community partners became community researchers, and when this became evident in the communities, several people in Alert Bay said to Vera, "It is so great to know it's our people doing the research." She understood this to signify that the overall meaningfulness and relevance of the study to community members would be enhanced by her leadership in the project.

The initial team had begun the project conversant with earlier drafts of the current CIHR guidelines (2004) and earlier drafts of the current OCAP principles (First Nations Centre 2007). However, the new academic team was committed to reconfiguring the RAMP as a full and complex partnership among Aboriginal community researchers and academic researchers, and to taking the historical and ongoing colonial context into account. We committed to being transparent, accountable, and reflexive in our relationships and conduct with all members of the team.

The project became a collaborative effort by Aboriginal women from the Nuxalk, Haida, and 'Namgis First Nations and academic researchers from the University of British Columbia in nursing, medicine, and counselling psychology. The new team used an ethnographic approach within a partici-patory framework. The community team members, women from each of the Aboriginal communities of Alert Bay, Bella Coola, Old Massett, and Skidegate, who wished to explore birthing issues in their communities, be-came "community researchers," both in name and role. Together, we studied Aboriginal women's experiences of traditional birthing practices and cur-rent maternity care, and their ideas and desires for future care.

The community researchers interviewed over a hundred women individ-ually or in focus groups, and they involved many more community mem-bers through informal interviews and community meetings. We conducted "fieldwork" in ways that drew on both ethnographic and Aboriginal trad-itions. The academic researchers from Vancouver spent time in the rural communities, and the entire team met in Vancouver and Alert Bay. We ana-lyzed interview and fieldwork data within each community and conducted an across-community analysis with all members of the academic and com-munity teams. In the process, both the community and academic research-ers learned as much about how to do research in the context of Aboriginal communities as we learned about rural maternity care. While each aspect of the research fostered meaningful participation of Aboriginal community members and researchers, we wish to emphasize the efforts that enhanced the capacity of the academic researchers to work with Aboriginal commun-ities and to follow indigenous scholars such as Smith (1999), Tenfingers (2005), Battiste and Henderson (2000), and Cole (2004) in an effort to question the very frameworks upon which our work often is based. Our work together drew attention to the contradiction between the rhetoric of "capacity building" as being *for* Aboriginal people and communities and the reality of our needs as academic researchers to develop our own capacities. Our analysis of these processes highlighted the critical importance of rela-tionships and reflexivity as method.

Whose Science? Whose Knowledge? Whose Methodology? Enhancing the Capacity of Academic Researchers to Work in Aboriginal Communities

Enhancing the capacity of academic researchers occurred in three broad interrelated areas involving questions regarding whose knowledge domin-ated, how leadership was enacted, and how resources were allocated. Throughout, analyses of language and power dynamics (among team mem-bers, within communities, and within society generally) were central to our examination of research practices. Analyses in these areas have implications for research methods and budgets that we believe are relevant not only to the conduct of research with Aboriginal people, but also to the ethical and effective conduct of research more generally.

We consider commitment to equitable and meaningful partnerships to be a moral imperative in working with Aboriginal people, particularly in light of the long history of exploitation of Aboriginal people through research, and the historical partnerships between colonial and academic interests. This moral imperative is not only towards mitigating harm but also towards harnessing research to redress harm in any way possible. Commitment to equitable partnerships has methodological implications in terms of who designs and guides the research, who participates, how decisions are made, how resources are used, how conflicts are identified and addressed, whose concerns dominate the work, how data are collected, who collects data, who analyses data and how, who disseminates findings and how, and how the data and findings are used and to whose benefit.

From the beginning of our work together, we had to struggle against multiple influences that conspired to privilege academics and academic Eurocentric knowledge over the community researchers and their knowledge. Although the academic team members had experience in community-based research and partnership-based research in Aboriginal communities, university and funding structures meant that the academics controlled the funds and controlled how the project would be carried out. Initially, the community researchers seemed to assume that the academics would retain control. However, as soon as the academic researchers indicated a willingness to be guided by the community researchers, they quickly offered direction. When the reconfigured team examined the previous budget, we talked about the meagre allocations for "honoraria":

> I was frustrated and embarrassed. I could not believe that the women had been put in the position of offering $10 as an honorarium for interviews. Not even enough to cover child care for the women. I was glad we brought it up though – Vera and Karen were also embarrassed, and quite relieved when we all decided that a more respectful amount would be offered. It seemed to me that after we made that decision, Vera brought up a number of problems with how the project had been done to this point. (CV, field notes, April 2005)

In the first year of the project, the community researchers primarily had been asked to provide community liaison, to recruit participants, and to gather data, but as the configuration of the team changed, their roles

rapidly expanded to include participation in all decision-making and research activities. The academic researchers intentionally tried to follow the
lead of the community researchers. Doing so meant that the community
researchers provided direction about how data would be collected, who
would collect the data, how they would be analyzed, and what constituted
data. Initially, this meant modifying the interview processes – for example,
shifting from semi-structured interviews to open-ended conversation. In
part, this shift aligned with the academic members of the new research team's
participatory and feminist orientation to qualitative research. It also stemmed
from the community researchers' clear understanding of what would work
in each community and what they felt competent and comfortable doing.
The community researchers take-up of leadership allowed for variation
among communities. For example, in one community, individual interviews
did not seem feasible, but focus groups worked very well; in other communities, the modified individual interview process was preferred.

Eventually, the leadership of the community researchers meant that what
constituted data and method was continuously questioned. For example, in
one community, the community researchers thought that reading and analysis of the transcripts should begin with the transcript of a focus group
with Elders. Beginning with what the community researchers called "the
wisdom of the Elders" provided an analytic background for the subsequent
inductive process used in reading other participant interviews and fieldwork data. In other communities, the academic researchers attended language classes, visited the ancestral homes of some of the researchers,
attended cultural events, participated in community ceremonies and activities, observed community members and Elders facilitating community
meetings and discussions, took part in traditional jewellery making, and so
on. This learning exemplified capacity building as a two-way street, as academics undertook to develop knowledge that the community researchers
thought would enhance the research. While the community researchers
learned skills such as interviewing, data analysis, presentation, and community action strategies through standard academic approaches such as
workshops, the academic researchers learned about history, culture, language, and themselves through listening to stories, songs, films, and language, and through experiencing the land and culture directly. From Vera's
perspective, our project formalized her "know-how" regarding how to ask
questions and really listen to the voices from her community, while also
paying her to do work she was already doing to strengthen her own culture

and community – taking it "beyond the kitchen table." Further, the community researchers from various First Nations learned about one another's culture, traditions, and history.

One of the most powerful examples of the two-way street in operation was the trip by the entire team to Village Island, Vera's ancestral village. Considering where and how we might learn about birthing experiences, the community researchers advised the trip. We chartered a fishing boat (idled by the collapse of the salmon fishery) to take the academic and community researchers from all four communities to this small island. Environmental and economic changes that made self-sufficiency untenable, coupled with the requirement to send children to residential school, led to Village Island now being uninhabited:

> The silence was full and heavy. Once Vera stopped drumming and we climbed out of the dinghy, we stepped into silence, profound but for the lapping waves and the occasional bird cry. Walking the island, seeing the downed totems half-buried in the grass, and hearing of Vera's childhood, I was saddened more deeply than I ever have been when reading historical accounts of the forced removal of people from their land. The workmanship, the beauty of the gates still standing speak of both the destruction and enduring spirits of the Kwakw<u>aka</u>'wakw people. (CV, field notes, May 2006)

> On leaving Village Island in the afternoon, I had a better sense of what a connection to a personal and cultural birthplace might feel like; it seemed important to ground the research we are doing together in the particular, unique, and palpable history and geography of the places we are invited to. The tide was running fast as we rowed in the dinghy back to the boat. As we motored back towards Cormorant Island, Vera said we might see a killer whale as she drummed. In about five minutes we saw to the south a black dorsal fin break the surface and a distant plume of vapour signal the killer whale's presence. It was as if she called it. Vera kept on drumming and singing. (BC, field notes, May 2006)

Continually asking "whose knowledge?" and "whose methodology?" required attending to every signal of discomfort expressed by the community researchers and knowing that these were important signals for the academic researchers to stop, question, and act differently. For example, when reading Betty's field notes above, Vera reminded the academic team about the potential to misread or misrepresent meanings of particular situations. She said:

The reason the whale came is because they are our family, we are all connected. I did not "call" the whale, as some might think. In our culture, there
is no calling because the connection is always there.

While, as a team of researchers we each bring our interpretive frames to our
experiences and the data, capacity building as a two-way street means listening carefully to our responses to one another's interpretations, and
at times, challenging the meaning ascribed. We do not believe there are
"wrong" interpretations, rather, that we have an obligation to scrutinize the
representations from our work together in ways that optimize our research
relationships and the relevance of our findings in their local contexts.

Being open to questioning what knowledge dominated helped us to
benefit from the research capacity that the community researchers *already*
had. For example, Vera questioned the original interview protocols, because she wanted a more narrative approach to the interviews, not a list of
academic-type questions. The power of who gets to ask was shifted by Vera's
questioning, "Do I have to use them? or could I just listen?" A participant in
another community had a similar experience. She was interviewed initially
using the interview guide developed by the original team, and what she perceived was an unfriendly interviewer, "trying to extract information" from
her. The process left her feeling shut down and angry. This experience led
her to taking a community researcher role, and learning how to do interviews in a "community-based way" that fit better with what she knew of
women in her community, who she also anticipated would not want to be
"interrogated" by a fly-in researcher. She spoke emphatically about her pref-
erence for listening to stories and allowing them to unfold in a respectful,
non-interruptive way, by avoiding a programmed or predetermined set of
questions and prompts. She thought that mixed focus groups, composed of
both youths and Elders, might allow a free flow of stories and ideas and a
sense of support and connection between community members in a way
that individual interviews would not. She subsequently conducted two
focus groups, one of which included young men, in which rich stories were
told. Women from each of the communities said in different ways that they
wanted to be interviewed by their own people because they would likely
speak more openly to a community member, and they might have greater
confidence that the research would be of significance and benefit to the
community.

Being open to evolving methods fostered the possibility of creating
"rigorous" research in the eyes of the community researchers and the

participants. Not only were data collection methods influenced; all aspects of method were scrutinized. For example, dissemination methods were significantly expanded beyond the usual academic routes, and these included casual encounters in coffee shops, being present at traditional dancing, presentations at community meetings, and informal meetings with leaders.

Leadership was not simply shifted from academic researchers to community researchers. Rather, leadership was thoughtfully considered, shared, and interrogated. We asked, who holds the pen? in figuring out who should record our emerging ideas on flip-chart paper. Together, we questioned whether the pen always trumps the tongue. The perceived power of the pen was attenuated when relations/power were negotiated in respectful ways that honoured the shared analysis that was underway. When Betty held the pen, it was after there was a sense that she would do it well – that is, everyone trusted she would represent the conversations and insights in ways that attended to power and language. Rather than controlling group process, she acted as a recorder and transcriber, trying to listen carefully and record the process and content of the group discussions, and then seeking input or correction from the group.

We also asked, who holds the purse? It was critically important to examine how people were paid, what was being paid for, and the extent to which the research could contribute to the local economy. Although we could not change the fact that the funds flowed through an academic organization, we made decisions about budget in an increasingly collective manner, as the new team coalesced. We worked within the constraints of the existing budget to try to pay people as respectfully and fairly as possible, and we hired local services as much as possible – for example, holding the final team meeting in Alert Bay, rather than Vancouver.

Explicitly naming capacity building as a "two-way street" shifted power relations in ways that enhanced our ability to create useful knowledge. In fact, we had to rethink and question dominant conventions about what "counts" as a useful research product itself. For example, while the academic researchers brought ideas about the importance of knowledge translation into deliberations about dissemination, the community researchers helped the team to see that any efforts to "translate" knowledge rely upon the very idea of what knowledge "is." The team agreed that knowledge from the research ought to make a difference in the everyday lives of people in the community, while the academic team brought a commitment to contributing to a larger body of knowledge about rural Aboriginal maternity care. The degree to which we could hold both purposes simultaneously relied upon the capacity of all to see how claims to knowledge and our methods of research are imbued with power relations. Yet, in our work together, power relations were viewed in the positive sense of expanding possibilities, challenging assumptions, and remaking our research practices in collaborative ways. Shifting our language to name the community partners as community researchers signalled power shifting from an academic core and community periphery to a more partnership-based model. This shift illustrates the importance of negotiated positioning in relation to the larger project of constructing useful knowledge at the community level. However, this shifting of power relations and related research processes was neither simply semantic nor token. Rather, the community researchers were able to build on relationships with participants, gather meaningful data in ways that suited the participants, ask locally relevant questions, and bring a wealth of contextual knowledge to the analysis. Participants shared their understandings and knowledge in very different ways than they would have with unfamiliar academic researchers. Several echoed the sentiment expressed in Alert Bay, saying, "We're glad it's *our* people doing the research."

This explicit stance of reciprocity assisted us to question all aspects of the research. For example, when one woman referred to research as "when they come and take our stories," together we turned that around to ask, "Who needs to hear these stories in your community, and among the policy makers?" signalling our rethinking of what might constitute knowledge translation processes.

Despite our attention to important issues and work to revise our practices accordingly, our processes were not flawless. We disagreed with one another, changed our minds about things, had tensions between various team members, and did not accomplish as much as we had hoped before the budget was expended. However, we produced what we think is a useful understanding of rural Aboriginal women's experiences of maternity care (Brown, Varcoe, and Calam, in press), and more importantly to us, completed the project with positive, respectful relationships. Our analysis of our experience suggests that thoughtful attention to the quality of the relationships between and among us all, and reflexivity on the part of individuals, was central to our approach to capacity building.

Reflexivity and Relationships as Methodology

Reflexivity was key to our research process – not as a process of navel gazing, but as a means to monitor our own actions and beliefs as participants in community-based research. As academic researchers we needed to examine continually how our varied privileges shaped our thinking and our relationships. For example, the academic researchers enjoyed relative affluence compared with the community researchers – questions such as, What is affordable? How are the community researchers being compensated? and so on, called into question our unearned privileges and how we continue to benefit from colonization.

We continuously had to question the extent to which the relationships we developed and the research processes we employed, such as trips to ancestral villages and participation in cultural events, were serving the community and knowledge development versus our own learning and enjoyment. We also repeatedly examined the consonance between our commitment to decolonizing values and our day-to-day behaviours within the team and in the participating communities. When reading the first draft of this chapter, Vera called attention to the tendency to talk "about" Aboriginal people in a text such as this in ways that further distinguish the "Other." How do we speak together in writing such as this to realize the very intent of this chapter? How could our writing practices embody the idea of leading and learning all at once? These questions serve as our ongoing challenges within the realm of participatory research.

Negotiating Meanings of Trust

Trust is an often-used concept in research relationships and seems integral to capacity building as we understand it. Our experiences illustrate how trust is never a given, but rather, is created through attention to relationships and reflexivity. In Vera's words, the new academic team "began in mistrust." From the inception of the new team, we worked to build and maintain trustworthy relationships. Rather than assuming that "good" relationships are static over time and place, we became aware that in each moment of research, our ways of being had to be trustworthy. That is, we had to continually negotiate new meanings of trust in the wake of history generally, and the specific history of the project. For example, during the circumstances that led to the team changeover, we sought guidance from both community and university authorities to help us address the conflict and attend to the ethical and relational issues among university team members. We consulted with an Aboriginal community researcher, Aboriginal Elders, academic participatory action researchers, the university equity office, and an ethicist to explore reparative actions that we could take. In particular, one Aboriginal consultant asked what it would take to conduct the research "in a good way" that would increase trust and not bring into the participating communities additional burdens or troubles created by academics. He cautioned against "keeping secrets" or withholding information from the community researchers or the communities themselves, and advised that we seek a solution that could keep the project functioning, but in an open, transparent, and effective way. As suggested earlier, several community researchers expressed feelings of exclusion from the communication and decision-making process concerning the academic team changeover. They stated that they were not informed either openly or in a timely manner. Unfortunately, the new team was caught up in the breakdown of relationships with the previous team members, and the timelines and ethical protocols at the university for resolving conflicts prevented the new team from dealing with the matter in a more open and expedient fashion.

The disruption in research relationships took time to surface. As a reconfigured team, we met with each community researcher in the spring following the changeover, and during a team gathering later that year to discuss face to face what had occurred, and to begin rebuilding our team relationships. Our intent was to discuss what was necessary to create trustworthy relationships with the new team, knowing that the disruption of the project provided the chance to remake relationships in ways that were honouring and respectful of power, history, and our shared hopes for improving maternity care in rural Aboriginal communities. Although it slowed the momentum of the project for a year, we deepened our awareness, and became attuned in a critical way to the importance of continually reflecting on how the values and principles of respect, relevance, reciprocity, and responsibility were neither static nor could be taken for granted in the name of "participatory" research. Rather, relationships had to be *experienced* as respectful and trustworthy and required continuous negotiation as the team changed. It required an open and non-defensive response to past harms experienced by the community researchers and academic team members prior to the team changeover. It also required time and resources for group and personal debriefing and ongoing relationship building.

Relationships could not be taken for granted in this context; rather, as co-researchers we continuously negotiated our relationships as partners at the level of each specific community and the wider project. For example, the community researcher who expressed concern about "keeping secrets" told us that her early childhood issues of trust and abandonment had resurfaced during the transition period. Issues of trust were also associated with some of the community researchers' own histories of trauma as survivors of the residential school system. Community researchers commented on the fact that they were able to express these concerns about trust and safety because they experienced openness on the part of the academic researchers to hear and validate their concerns. While several thought that trust had been "re-established" with the new team, they continued to caution that building trust requires time and ongoing attention. Relationships evolved throughout the project and sustained the team through to completion and into new collaborations.

Implications: Building Capacity as a Two-Way Street

Overall, the academic researchers came to more fully appreciate how expanding notions of capacity as a two-way street required a willingness to continuously negotiate the complex web of research relationships as they are shaped by history, context, and power relations. Capacity building as a two-way street also required interrogating conventional research practices to realize our decolonizing intent. Because our intent was to create knowledge that could enhance birthing experiences for the women in the four communities, and ongoing colonial relations were identified as shaping rural health care delivery in several communities, it follows that our methodological processes warranted the same critical scrutiny as our emerging findings. Our capacity being enhanced, however, is not the end of the story, so to speak. Capacity building must be both a means and an end all at once, assisting us to contribute to the larger aims of reducing and redressing inequity; democratizing research; preventing domination, exploitation, and suffering; and interrogating conventional methodological concepts and practice approaches that further colonial domination.

From our analysis of our experiences, we think that the following principles might guide capacity building when doing research within Aboriginal communities:

- Continuously question Eurocentric assumptions regarding what is considered to be legitimate knowledge and methods.
- Scrutinize the historical context of research in local settings.
- Begin decolonizing methodologies by working to develop decolonizing relationships.

- Follow indigenous leadership.
- Take direction from indigenous knowledge and local knowledge and traditions.
- Reconceptualize knowledge translation from indigenous and local standpoints.
- Develop "indigenous" criteria for guiding and evaluating research.

Implications for Academic Researchers

Following these principles means that academic researchers, including Aboriginal academic researchers, must assume the stance of learner. Learning from the appropriate people in Aboriginal communities – Elders, community leaders, research participants – requires an orientation of openness and inquiry. Rather than positioning oneself as an "expert," humility and a willingness to learn are needed. Critical self-reflection is a hallmark of feminist research, but crossing the multiple "differences" occasioned by colonizing processes – experiences of poverty, racism, access to education, and so on – requires an intense level of self-reflection: examining biases, assumptions, projections, and our own identities. Such questioning is unending – those of us in the role of academic researcher didn't "get it" in some enlightened way; rather, the need for always assuming a stance of unknowing and willingness to learn was reaffirmed.

Academic researchers must learn and further their abilities to listen and participate in groups in new ways. Some of these new ways arise out of particular cultural norms for listening and speaking that vary with different Aboriginal communities. Some arise from the dynamics occasioned by a group of people with diverse perspectives attempting to generate new knowledge and create equitable conditions for doing so collaboratively in the context of multiple differences, including differences of power and privilege.

Implications for Method

Methods that seek to build capacity in academic researchers and community-based Aboriginal researchers must incorporate learning about the histories and culture of the people involved – particularly pre-colonial histories, the history of colonizing, and how these histories shape everyone's lives today. We would now begin any project with "workshops" about history and culture as well as about interviewing and analysis techniques. We would take direction from Aboriginal partners as to where we should begin – perhaps Elders, storytellers, or community leaders.

If capacity building truly is to be a two-way street, then methodology should be seen as an enactment of indigenous knowledge and practice. As academics, we learned how to follow better, and how to control less. One good example was when one community researcher asked in preparation for leading her first group interview, "What do I do with these focus group questions?" Our answer, "Keep them in your back pocket, you will know the questions to ask," suggests that we had loosened some rigid notions of rigour that our research training might have instilled.

Finally, measures and resources for developing and continuously examining trustworthy research relationships among and between all participants are required. Seeking understanding about group dynamics and conflict resolution, and devoting time and resources to getting to know and understand one another, should be legitimate components of the research timeline, and a priority throughout.

Implications for Research Budgets

Power relations and what is valued can be seen in research budgets. How people are paid, for example, shows whose knowledge and whose methods are valued. We think that pay equity should recognize indigenous knowledge. Further, practices regarding offering honoraria to recognize various forms of research participation should be questioned and approaches developed in consultation with local communities. Wherever possible, opportunities for meaningful employment should be planned. Budgets should explicitly include resources for opportunities for all to learn about particular histories that cannot be learned from written (and often Eurocentric) accounts, and include resources for learning from oral history and experiential learning. Finally, budgeting should allocate time and resources for interpersonal debriefing and guidance for optimizing team dynamics.

Implications for Research Organizations

The language and underlying assumptions used by funding bodies and ethics-monitoring bodies should explicitly recognize capacity building as a two-way street. Aboriginal people should be recognized and compensated for contributing their knowledge and leadership. Guidelines should be fundamentally informed by indigenous perspectives. Academic researchers, particularly non-Aboriginal researchers, should take the lead from Aboriginal partners, continuously striving to "work themselves out of a job." Aboriginal organizations should continue to demand more complex, reciprocal relationships in research.

Conclusion

Tenfingers asserts that "First Nations people in Canada and the world are increasingly rejecting Western, colonial frameworks of research and policy development. Instead, we are reclaiming our right to be who we are, and we are revitalizing our cultures through promotion and utilization of indigenous research methodologies and development of culturally-rooted policy" (2005, S60). Academic researchers can support, participate in, and learn from this movement with conscious and open negotiation of relationships, and reflexivity about interpersonal and group power dynamics and their impact on the research process. In both Aboriginal and non-Aboriginal contexts, capacity building must be a two-way endeavour if research is to be relational, decolonizing, and anti-racist.

ACKNOWLEDGMENTS
This chapter draws on the Rural Aboriginal Maternity Care Project, funded by CIHR and completed by Laura Bell (Old Massett), Myrna Bell Wilson (Old Massett), Helen Brown (UBC), Marla Buchanan (UBC), Betty Calam (UBC), Karen Cook (Alert Bay), Barb Cranmer (Alert Bay), Melissa Edgars (Skidegate), Jen Eskes (UBC), Thelma Harvey (Bella Coola), Vera Newman (Alert Bay), Miranda Tallio (Bella Coola), Jen Valentine (UBC), Colleen Varcoe (UBC), and Mary Ann Wilson (Skidegate).

REFERENCES
Battiste, M., and J. Youngblood Henderson. 2000. *Protecting Indigenous Knowledge and Heritage*. Saskatoon, SK: Purich.

Brown, H., C. Varcoe, and B. Calam. In press. "Engaging Nurses in Health Promoting Rural Aboriginal Maternity Care in a Neo-Colonial Canadian Context." *Canadian Journal of Nursing Research*.

Brown, M. 2005. "Research, Respect and Responsibility: A Critical Review of the Tri-Council Policy Statement in Aboriginal Community-Based Research." *Pimatisiwin: A Journal of Aboriginal and Indigenous Community Health* 3(2): 79-100.

CIHR (Canadian Institutes of Health Research). 2004. Capacity-Building Workshops (Archived Request for Applications), HIV/AIDS Community-Based Research Program. Available at http://www.cihr-irsc.gc.ca/e/25189.html.

–. 2007. *CIHR Guidelines for Health Research Involving Aboriginal People*. Available at http://www.cihr-irsc.gc.ca/e/29134.html.

Cole, P. 2004. "Trick(ster)s of Aboriginal Research: Or How to Use Ethical Review Strategies to Perpetuate Cultural Genocide." *Native Studies Review* 15(2): 7-36.

Cook, E.-D., and D. Howe. 2004. "Aboriginal Languages of Canada." In W.O'Grady and J. Archibald, eds. *Contemporary Linguistic Analysis*, 294-309. Toronto: Addison-Wesley Longman.

Eikeland, O. 2006. "Condescending Ethics and Action Research." *Action Research* 4(1): 37-47.

First Nations Centre. 2007. *OCAP: Ownership, Control, Access and Possession.* Sanctioned by the First Nations Information Governance Committee, Assembly of First Nations. Ottawa: National Aboriginal Health Organization.

Fiske, J. 1995. "Political Status of Native Indian Women: Contradictory Implications of Canadian State Policy." *American Indian Culture and Research Journal* 19(2): 1-30.

—. 2000. "By, For, or About? Shifting Directions in the Representations of Aboriginal Women." *Atlantis* 25(1): 11-27.

—. 2006. "Boundary Crossings: Power and Marginalisation in the Formation of Canadian Aboriginal Women's Identities." *Gender and Development* 14(2): 247-58.

Fiske, J., and A.J. Browne. 2004. *First Nations Women and the Paradox of Health Policy Reform.* Vancouver: BC Centre of Excellence for Women's Health.

Interagency Advisory Panel on Research Ethics. 2008. *Draft 2nd Edition of the Tri-Council Policy Statement: Ethical Conduct for Research Involving Humans.* Ottawa: Interagency Secretariat on Research Ethics.

Smith, D.G., ed. 1974. *The Adventures and Sufferings of John R. Jewitt, Captive among the Nootka, 1803-1805.* Toronto: McClelland and Stewart.

Smith, Linda Tuhiwai. 1999. *Decolonizing Methodologies: Research and Indigenous People.* London: Zed Books.

Tenfingers, K. 2005. "Rejecting, Revitalizing, and Reclaiming: First Nations Work to Set the Direction of Research and Policy Development." *Canadian Journal of Public Health* 96(Jan./Feb.): S60-S63.

13

Reflections
Promises and Limits of Feminist
Community Research

GILLIAN CREESE AND WENDY FRISBY

This collection grapples, in different ways, with both the promises and limitations of feminist community research. If we expect feminist approaches to collaborative research with diverse communities to resolve power inequalities between researchers and community participants, we are bound to be disappointed. As post-structuralist feminists have argued, reflexivity may make us more conscious of hierarchies of positionality and marginalization, but it is naive to suggest that it alone will resolve such differences (Houle 2009; Stacey 1988; Visweswaran 1994). It is in naming and providing alternatives to the conditions that create social inequalities that the strength of feminist community research lies. At the same time, feminist critiques of contested, multiple, and partial interests, experiences, perspectives, and "truths" in the research process apply to feminist methodologies, too. However, we argue that researchers can negotiate research relationships in ways that have the potential to be *more rather than less equitable*, and the case studies in this collection contribute in important ways to that larger enterprise.

The promise of feminist community research is not that these methods can produce full (rather than partial) accounts of the social world untainted by ongoing hierarchies of power and privilege that are tied to gender, racialization, social class, sexuality, age, (dis)ability, and so on. Instead, the promise lies in the ongoing and continual learning from previous studies about what works better in what contexts, including what compromises might be made (and what cannot be compromised), with what consequences and for whom, in order to attain more equal forms of reflexive community collaboration. More collaborative and equitable conditions of knowledge creation, we believe, have the potential to expand our understandings in new directions and, hence, contribute to social change by revealing the consequences of inequality and exploring alternative approaches for ameliorating or at least lessening them. The wide range of empirical case studies in this collection, and the commitment to detailing failings as well as accomplishments, provide instructive examples for other researchers who are interested in continuing to move forward in this collective project.

The case studies emphasize the importance of negotiating relationships in order to conduct research with, rather than "on" or "for," identifiable groups that are diverse rather than homogeneous. Negotiation requires much more than top-down consultation, and is most effective the earlier it begins and the longer it continues in the research process. Although negotiating research relationships rarely occurs among equals (given different social locations and regimes of funding, for example), procedures that are collectively developed and employed can either enhance or limit possibilities for power sharing. As these case studies illustrate, the more flexible and reflexive the research design, the more power sharing is facilitated in processes of collaborative knowledge construction. Engaging in community collaboration to define research questions, what constitutes data, procedures for data collection and resource allocation, and strategies of meaning making enhance possibilities for trust and more equal research partnerships. Of course, as many case studies in this volume indicate, optimal collaboration at every stage of research cannot always be realized, given constraints of geography and time, funding requirements, approval boards, the nature of community engagement, and other contingencies. So, although the focus on collaboration through negotiation remains distinctive from conventional research in social sciences, health care, education, and other disciplines, the levels of power sharing accomplished vary considerably and must be taken into account when making knowledge claims.

More equitable collaborations emanate from negotiations that are both transparent and ongoing throughout the research process, although this ideal form of collaboration is not always easily attained. Several studies in this collection did develop mechanisms for continuous (re)negotiation during the research process (particularly chapters 5, 9, and 12, where community/peer researchers were central to the process), while others confronted significant institutional barriers to adopting the desires of community partners when funders or other approval agencies had divergent demands or goals (e.g., chapters 7, 10, and 11). Other chapters point to the problem of unmet expectations, either by promising more than researchers can deliver (such as change in government policies or social conditions) or facing different sets of expectations among community participants, between community participants and researchers, or among different members of the research team (e.g., chapters 2, 3, and 4). These divergent outcomes remind us that research is always socially embedded in a multitude of institutional structures and social relations that can have an impact on what it is possible to accomplish in a given context.

As all the case studies in this collection demonstrate, developing an understanding of the historical, institutional, and material contexts in which the research communities are located is critical for developing more equitable research relationships. This is so whether engaged in research within local Canadian, diasporic, or international contexts, with communities to which we are (at least partial) "insiders," or those whose social locations have less in common with the researchers. Without a sound grasp of historical, institutional, and material conditions, and how community participants differentially make sense of them, researchers are less likely to actively hear or understand what participants are telling them, which, in turn, is less likely to generate findings that have relevance to the communities within which they work. Indeed, this book provides many examples of both the possibilities and the importance of this kind of "two-way learning" that unsettles patronizing dichotomies between "expert" researchers and less knowledgeable/capable community participants (e.g., chapters 4, 5, 6, 10, and 12). More equitable collaborations rest on recognizing that community participants have much to teach academic researchers in ways that cannot always be anticipated, the content of which may not always be appreciated if it contradicts the researcher's own aims, social locations, or assumptions.

From the beginning, the authors in this collection set out to expose problems and limitations in feminist community research, as much as sharing creative solutions and accomplishments, in order to encourage advancements in FCR, rather than to position their own work as a sort of panacea. Although all begin from a series of feminist methodological principles about conducting ethical, reflexive, collaborative, and change-oriented research, in one way or another every chapter also broaches the practicalities of compromise, where idealism meets the "real world" of social research, as necessary parts of the research process. Hence, throughout this text, the limits of reflexivity are as evident as its efficacy. Learning to compromise in terms of expectations of feminist collaborations, and weighing what is and is not compromisable, is part of the real practice of this type of research. For several authors in this collection, for example, funding arrangements highlighted the limits of reciprocity, making it difficult or impossible to give up financial control (and, here, Chapter 9 is the exception), although most found more creative ways to redistribute resources than is typical in conventional research, including the time needed to build at least some level of trust as a basis for building university/community relationships.

In the introductory chapter, we alluded to the policy implications of the studies in this collection, a topic that deserves specific attention in a future volume dedicated to feminist community research. As an initial step, some of the case studies analyzed here were closely tied to government policies through funding sources or research designed for policy evaluation, which made it more difficult for community partners to redefine questions and approaches (see chapters 3, 7, 8, and 10). The double-sided nature of such compromises is apparent in the case of development work, for example, where "gender mainstreaming," embedded in assumptions of funders and local community leaders, threatened to depoliticize feminist research, while also opening up spaces for local women to assume new leadership positions (see chapter 3). Alternatively, possibilities exist for including policy makers who see the potential relevance of feminist community research as a way to foster social change, given the institutional barriers they encounter (see chapter 6). While this approach has many potential pitfalls, the possibilities for collaborating with policy makers who are "on board" have not yet been fully explored.

The contributors in this volume are engaged in feminist community research as part of a broader commitment to social change. These case studies all surface often silenced knowledge linked to marginalized groups (including sex workers, women in prison, recent immigrants, women on social assistance, and Aboriginal mothers), and in so doing, they can help to facilitate broader long-term initiatives to enhance social justice. Several authors explicitly address immersion in political processes, documenting explicit state interference in research (as in chapter 10), or redefining the research process as "an intervention" (in chapter 5), or as "political work" (in chapter 7). The project of decolonizing knowledge identified by many authors (especially chapters 2, 3, 6, 9, and 12) is inherently political, as is the overall feminist project that deconstructs the "neutral" (affluent male white Eurocentric positivist) research lens. Far from undercutting the credibility of research in this collection, acknowledgments of social location and broader social goals enhance the transparency of research processes by stripping away the veneer of unlocated disinterested objectivity that Donna Haraway evocatively calls the "god trick" (1991). Reflexively acknowledging social location and its impact on knowledge creation is critical for generating more equitable collaborations with communities, however the *community* is defined. Acknowledging and consciously working across differences does not mean that unequal power relations disappear, but it does form a more fruitful starting point for negotiating more genuine and egalitarian forms of collaboration in the production of knowledge. A central problem that remains, however, is how to convince various levels of government, particularly with the ascendance of neo-liberalism, that socially located research can and should inform social policies in ways that empower rather than disadvantage marginalized groups. The promise of feminist community research lies in producing knowledge that has empowering potentials for social change. The efficacy of feminist policy interventions in a neo-liberal era urgently awaits further examination so that in the end hope can supersede disappointment.

REFERENCES

Haraway, Donna. 1991. "Situated Knowledges: The Science Question in Feminism and the Privilege of Partial Perspectives." In *Simians, Cyborgs, and Women: The Reinvention of Nature*, 183-201. New York: Routledge.

Houle, Karen. 2009. "Making Strange: Deconstruction and Feminist Standpoint Theory." *Frontiers: A Journal of Women Studies* 30(1): 72-93.

Stacey, Judith. 1988. "Can There Be a Feminist Ethnography?" *Women's Studies International Forum* 11(1): 21-27.

Visweswaran, Kamala. 1994. "Betrayal: An Analysis in Three Acts." In Inderpal Grewal and Caren Kaplan, eds., *Scattered Hegemonies: Postmodernity and Transnational Feminist Practices*, 90-109. Minneapolis: University of Minnesota Press.

Contributors

Shari Allinott is a peer facilitator with the Maka Project and a co-director of Downtown Eastside Sex Workers United Against Violence. She is a former board member of PIVOT Legal Society and an outreach worker with several agencies, including Downtown Eastside Women's Centre.

Joan M. Anderson is a professor emerita at the University of British Columbia, and founding director of the Culture, Gender, and Health Research Unit in UBC's School of Nursing. Herself an immigrant woman of Colour, she has been doing research with immigrants of Colour, as well as with Canadian-born people of European descent, over the course of her research career. She has collaborated with health care agencies about getting these research findings into practice.

Leonora C. Angeles is an associate professor of community and regional planning and women's and gender studies at the University of British Columbia. She is also a faculty research associate of the Centre for Human Settlements and of the Centre for Southeast Asian Research. She has done community-based research in the Philippines, Vietnam, Thailand, Brazil, and Canada, particularly with women, farmers and fisherfolk, immigrant groups, local governments, and international solidarity networks.

Kashmir Besla works as a family counsellor with the Children's Foundation in Vancouver, British Columbia. Her work is primarily in the area of child protection concerns. Through the BC Schizophrenia Society, she facilitates groups for children who have a parent with mental illness, and she also works with men who are involved in the criminal justice system. She enjoys working on research projects and was a community-based researcher in the Women's Employability and Health Project.

Helen Brown is an assistant professor in the School of Nursing at the University of British Columbia. Her research interests in women's health and maternal infant care are focused on social justice, inequities, and health outcomes.

Marla J. Buchanan is an associate professor in the Department of Educational and Counselling Psychology and Special Education in the Faculty of Education at the University of British Columbia. She is currently the deputy head of her department. Her research interests include studies on traumatic stress among various populations and social justice issues (e.g., trauma in the culture of journalism, Aboriginal maternity care, women in prison). She teaches clinical supervision and advanced qualitative research methods in the Counselling Psychology Program.

Shauna Butterwick is an associate professor of adult education in the Department of Educational Studies at the University of British Columbia. Her research has focused on issues of social justice, most particularly women's learning in a variety of contexts (at work, in welfare programs, within social movements). She is also interested in arts-based processes and participatory and action-oriented inquiry, and their contributions to teaching and research on matters of social justice.

Bette Calam is an associate professor in the Department of Family Practice in the Faculty of Medicine at the University of British Columbia. Her scholarly work integrates community-based research and teaching, Aboriginal women's health, and medical education.

Katharine Chan is an MSc. student in the Faculty of Science (Biomedical Physiology and Kinesiology) at Simon Fraser University and a research project assistant with BC Cancer Agency in cancer control research and family and community oncology. She is also a research assistant for the BC Centre of Excellence for Women's Health with a focus on female smoking behaviour. In 2008-9, she worked as a research assistant for the Maka Project, a community partnership between WISH Drop-In Centre Society and the BC Centre for Excellence in HIV/AIDS. Her research interests include population health promotion and the prevention of disease, specifically through screening and social interventions.

Jill Chettiar has worked in a variety of non-profit and research positions in the Downtown Eastside of Vancouver since 1998. She worked as volunteer coordinator for the Vancouver Area Network of Drug Users in 2002-3 and as research coordinator for the North American Opiate Medication Initiative (NAOMI) in 2005-8. Currently, she is providing administrative support for the Sex Workers United Against Violence Society and working as project coordinator for the AESHA (An Evaluation of Sex Workers Health Access) Project.

Gillian Creese is the director of the Centre for Women's and Gender Studies and a professor in the Department of Sociology at the University of British Columbia. Her research interests include women and trade unions, feminist research methods, and immigration and settlement issues in Canada, with a special focus on the experiences of immigrant and refugee women from sub-Saharan Africa.

Adrian Fox is a peer facilitator with the Maka Project and a peer outreach worker with the Mobile Access Project (MAP) van for street-based sex workers. She is also a board member with the WISH Drop-In Centre Society.

Wendy Frisby is past chair of the Women's and Gender Studies program and a professor in the School of Human Kinetics at the University of British Columbia. She is also the co-director of the UBC Centre for Sport and Sustainability. She has been working with diverse collaborators on feminist participatory action research projects for over fifteen years and teaches courses in organizational theory, health promotion, and qualitative research methods.

Tara Gibb is a doctoral student in the Department of Educational Studies at the University of British Columbia. Her research focuses on adult education policy, with a current interest in adult second and/or additional language education policies in Canadian contexts.

Kate Gibson is the executive director of the WISH Drop-In Centre Society, a long-standing community organization whose mission is to increase the health, safety, and well-being of women working in the survival sex trade in Vancouver. In her role, she is responsible for the oversight of all programming associated with WISH, including fundraising and program development. Additional responsibilities include the promotion of initiatives that address the issues of poverty, health, discrimination, violence, and exclusion of women working on the street.

Penny Gurstein is the director of and a professor in the School of Community and Regional Planning at the University of British Columbia. Her research interests are in the socio-cultural aspects of community planning, with particular emphasis on those who are the most marginalized in planning processes.

Louise Hara is a community coach who has a strong interest in advancing the role of community-based research as a tool for transformative change. She is currently building a practice in partnership focused on strengthening the capacity of groups and communities to "become the change they want to see in the world." She acted as project coordinator on the Women's Employability and Health Project.

Evelyn Hamdon is a doctoral student in the Department of Educational Policy Studies at the University of Alberta; her research focus is on representations of Arab and Muslim women in popular culture. Currently, she is also the project coordinator for Global Citizenship Curriculum Development at the University of Alberta.

Xin Huang recently completed her PhD in the Centre for Women's and Gender Studies at the University of British Columbia. Her research focuses on gender and sexuality as well as issues related to culture, state, and society in contemporary China. Her doctoral research examines the legacy of the Maoist gender ideology in post-Mao China. She was a research assistant on the Multiculturalism and Physical Activity Project.

Paul Kershaw is the two-time recipient (2005, 2007) of the Jill Vickers Prize, awarded by the Canadian Political Science Association in recognition of outstanding scholarship about gender and politics. He is an assistant professor at the University of British Columbia in the College for Inter-disciplinary Studies and the Human Early Learning Partnership (HELP), where he is the HELP scholar in social care, citizenship, and the determin-ants of health; the director of the Social Care and Social Citizenship Research Network; and co-director of the Early Learning and Child Care Research Unit.

Edith Ngene Kambere is a social worker at Riverview Hospital in Metro Vancouver, British Columbia. For many years, she has been involved in de-veloping programs for African immigrant and refugee women and children. She is also a community activist, researcher, and a founding member of Umoja Operation Compassion Society/African Family Services, which pro-vides settlement services to immigrants and refugees from sub-Saharan Africa.

Connie Kaweesi is the chair of the Academic and Career Technology Programs at Northern Lights College in Dawson Creek, British Columbia. She is a social worker educator and has worked in the social and health care field for more than twenty-five years. She is the community-based research-er for the Women's Employability and Health Project. Her primary research interests include women's issues in northern communities, with a focus on women's health.

Koushambhi Basu Khan is the research manager of the Critical Research in Health and Healthcare Inequities unit in the School of Nursing at the Uni-versity of British Columbia. Her research interests and publications are in the area of culture and health, post-colonial feminism, ethnographic research, gender, poverty and health, immigrant population, and social suffering.

Robin LeDrew is a family support worker with Whitevalley Community Resource Centre in the rural village of Lumby, British Columbia. Her inter-ests in feminism, social justice, and community development have involved her in experimental communal living in the 1970s, organizing a re-evaluation counselling community in the North Okanagan in the 1980s and 1990s, the National Action Committee for the Status of Women in the early 1990s, and more recently, community-based research for the Women's Employability and Health Project.

Ruth Elwood Martin is a Vancouver Foundation community-based clinician investigator, a clinical professor at the University of British Columbia, the inaugural director of the Collaborating Centre for Prison Health and Education, the lead faculty member for research in the family medicine residency program, and a fellow of the College of Family Physicians of Canada. She has worked part-time as a family physician in prison medical clinics since 1994. Her academic interests include participatory research, primary care research, cervical cancer screening, women's health, and narrative medicine. In 2005, she engaged with women inside prison in a participatory health research project that continues in the community as Women In2 Healing.

Kelly Murphy, while incarcerated, in 2005, began participation in the Women In2 Healing research project, which seeks to collaborate with women as they are being released into the community to improve their health outcomes during that process. As a woman who has arisen out of abuse and adversity, she is now passionately involved in helping other women find their voice and rise up out of their own oppressive circumstances. Working with narratives and dialogue, she focuses on telling the stories of the women that she journeys with. She is the interview coordinator on the Doing Time Project at UBC. She also works as a community-based peer researcher with Women In2 Healing and Doing Time.

Vera Newman is a member of the 'Namgis Band and a project leader and researcher for several health research projects in Alert Bay, British Columbia. She is married to Chief Edwin Newman and has four grown children and five grandchildren. She is a member of a cultural group in Alert Bay that teaches and empowers people to be strong in their cultural heritage. She describes her grandchildren as her *Kwalayu*, meaning her purpose for living.

Devi Parsad was the project nurse with the Maka Project at the BC Centre for Excellence in HIV/AIDS, 2006-8, when she was also a community nurse with Insite in Vancouver. She has extensive experience as a community nurse with marginalized and HIV-affected populations in rural, as well as urban, BC communities. She is currently living in Prince George, where she works as a nurse and clinical instructor with the University of Northern British Columbia, while pursuing her MPH with the Centre for International Health at Curtin University in Western Australia.

Pamela Ponic is a postdoctoral fellow at the School of Nursing, University of British Columbia, and a community-based researcher with the BC Centre of Excellence in Women's Health. Her doctoral research involved a critical examination of social inclusion as a strategy for promoting health and community-based research with a group of women living in poverty. She was a research consultant on the Women's Employability and Health Project. Her passion is "bridging the gap" between the academy and community-based organizations and understanding all the complexities that accompany this crossing.

Jane Pulkingham is a professor of sociology and chair of the Department of Sociology and Anthropology at Simon Fraser University. Her research interests are in critical policy studies, focusing on gender and the state, welfare state restructuring and inequality, women and income security, and poverty studies.

Colleen Reid is a faculty member in Child, Family and Commmunity Studies at Douglas College, an adjunct professor at Simon Fraser University, and a research associate at the Centre for Women's and Gender Studies at the University of British Columbia. She is author of *The Wounds of Exclusion: Poverty, Women's Health and Social Justice* and co-author of *Experience, Research, Social Change: Methods beyond the Mainstream*. In her postdoctoral research, she was principal investigator of the Women's Employability and Health Project. Her work focuses on the social determinants of health, health inequalities, gender and health, community development, and feminist and community-based research methods.

Sheryl Reimer-Kirkham is an associate professor at Trinity Western University in Langley, British Columbia, where she teaches health care ethics in the Master of Arts in Leadership Program and in the Department of Nursing. Her scholarship is focused on culture, diversity, social justice, and health services. A current funded research project examines religious and spiritual plurality in health care. She is a founding member of TWU's new Religion in Canada Institute, TWU's Gender Studies Institute, and an investigator with the Culture, Gender, and Health Research Unit at the University of British Columbia. She has authored numerous peer-reviewed manuscripts and her dissertation was awarded the Governor General's Gold Medal at the University of British Columbia.

Kate Shannon is an assistant professor in the Faculty of Medicine (Division of AIDS) at the University of British Columbia and a research scientist with the BC Centre for Excellence in HIV/AIDS. She currently leads a five-year study, funded by the Canadian Institutes of Health Research, evaluating the impact of social and structural interventions targeting female sex workers on sexual health and vulnerability to HIV/STI infection. Her research program focuses on the social and structural dynamics (e.g., poverty and legislation of women's rights) of HIV/AIDS among women in Canada and globally, particularly in sub-Saharan Africa.

Mark W. Tyndall is the program director in epidemiology at the BC Centre for Excellence in HIV/AIDS. He is an associate professor in the Department of Medicine at the University of British Columbia and head of the Infectious Diseases Division at Providence Health Care. He has national and international research expertise in the area of clinical epidemiology, sexually transmitted infections, HIV/AIDS prevention and harm reduction, and HIV and Hepatitis C treatment among marginalized populations.

Colleen Varcoe is a professor in the School of Nursing at the University of British Columbia. Her program of research on violence and inequity examines women's health, with an emphasis on violence against women and Aboriginal women's health, and ethical nursing practice with an emphasis on cultural safety.

Silvia Vilches has been looking at the depletion of women's social and supportive networks through the changes in social assistance policy. She is also interested in rural community health and early childhood services capacity-development models, including ways of working cross-culturally to support capacity development in Aboriginal communities. Her four key interests are poverty, cross-cultural community development, the nexus of policy to practice, and gender.

Index

Printed and bound in Canada by Friesens

Set in Futura Condensed and Warnock by Artegraphica Design Co. Ltd.

Copy Editor: Kate Baltais

Proofreader: Lesley Erickson

Cartographer: Eric Leinberger

Indexer: Annette Lorek